PROFESSOR GRANT BRINKWORTH AND DR PENNIE TAYLOR

THE CSIRO
LOW-CARB
DIABETES
DIET & LIFESTYLE
SOLUTION

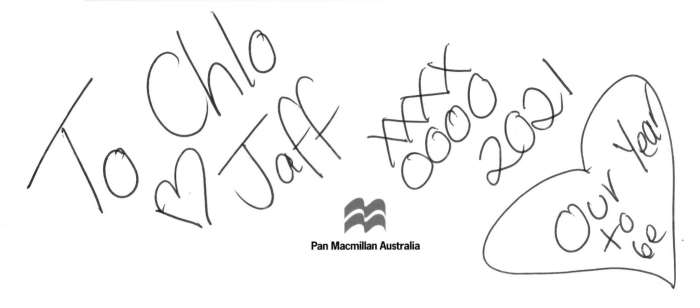

To Chlo
♥ Jaff
xxxx ooooo 2021
Our Year
xo be

Pan Macmillan Australia

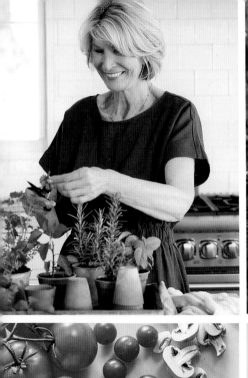
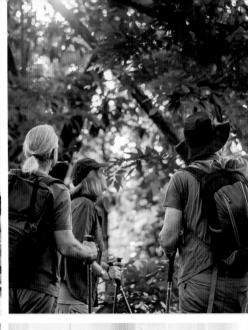
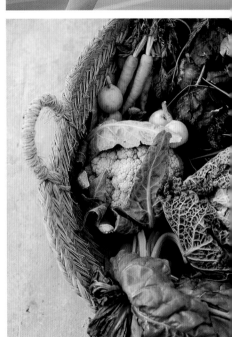
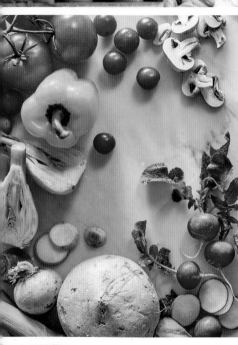
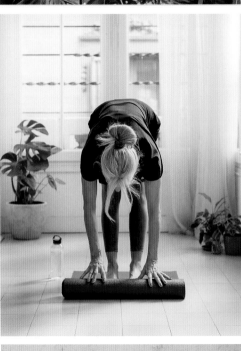
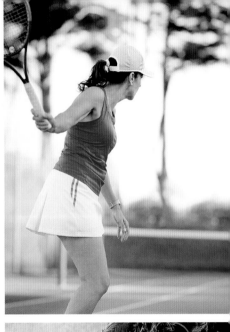
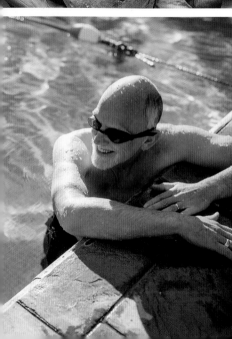
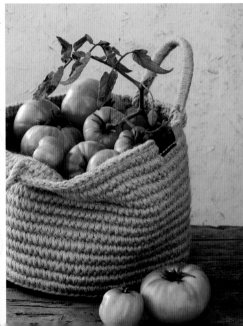
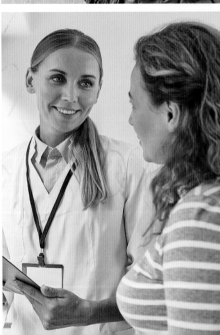

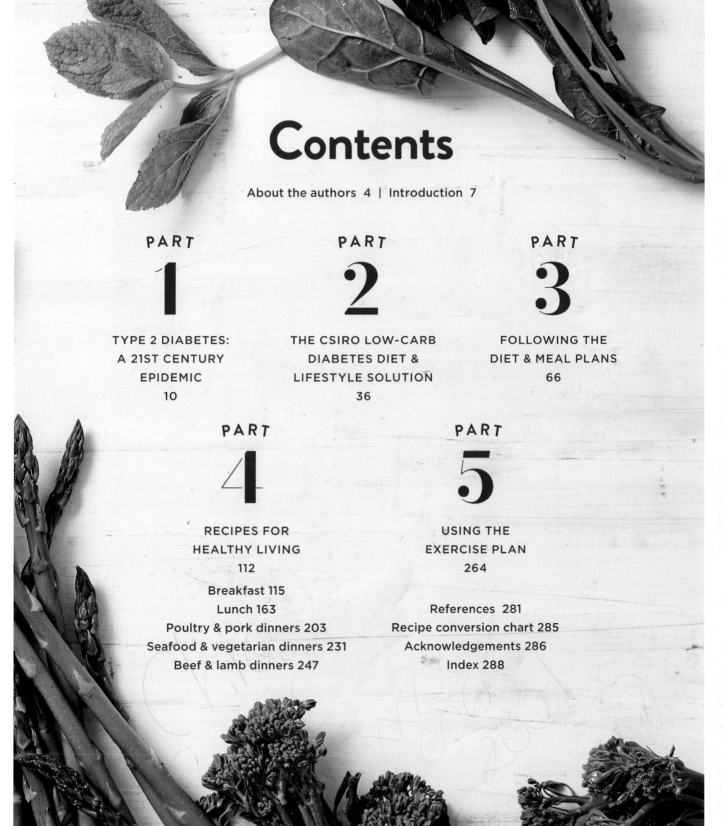

Contents

About the authors

PROFESSOR GRANT BRINKWORTH

Professor Grant Brinkworth is a Senior Principal Research Scientist at CSIRO – Health and Biosecurity. He has a PhD in nutrition science and exercise physiology and more than 20 years' experience leading large-scale clinical studies evaluating the effects of diets, foods, exercise and lifestyle interventions on human health, performance and functionality in healthy and clinical populations. Professor Brinkworth's research interests include developing, testing and translating effective nutrition, lifestyle and technology solutions for the management of obesity, metabolic health and type 2 diabetes and understanding the role of lower-carbohydrate dietary patterns for health and disease-risk management. He has published over 100 scientific papers and is the co-author of the number-one bestselling book *The CSIRO Low-carb Diet*, as well as *CSIRO Low-carb Every Day*, *CSIRO Low-carb Diet Quick & Easy* and *CSIRO Protein Plus*. Professor Brinkworth is an Adjunct Research Professor at the University of South Australia and Research Affiliate with the University of Sydney, and has supervised more than 10 post-graduate students in the areas of nutrition, exercise and metabolism. Professor Brinkworth also has a Master of Business Administration degree with strong interests in innovation and the commercialisation of science outcomes, technologies and lifestyle programs for large-scale community adoption and impact.

DOCTOR PENNIE TAYLOR

Dr Pennie Taylor is an Accredited Practising Dietitian (APD) and Research Scientist at CSIRO – Health and Biosecurity. She has a PhD from the University of Adelaide, School of Medicine exploring dietary factors and the integrated role of emerging health technologies including Real Time Continuous Glucose Monitoring (RT-CGM) for obesity and type 2 diabetes and lifestyle management. With more than 20 years' experience working in the health and research industry, she has extensive clinical nutrition expertise in diet and specialised food design for complex clinical trials and the development of community weight management and chronic disease programs, specialising in obesity, type 2 diabetes and metabolic weight-loss surgery. Dr Taylor has published over 30 peer-reviewed scientific papers and is co-author of the number-one bestselling book *The CSIRO Low-carb Diet*, as well as *CSIRO Low-carb Every Day*, *CSIRO Low-carb Diet Quick & Easy* and *CSIRO Healthy Gut Diet*. Dr Taylor works closely with industry and government partners to translate science into clinical and community outcomes with strong interests in utilising diabetes technology and novel foods for optimising self-management strategies for improved health and wellbeing across all life and health stages. Dr Taylor continues to practise privately at EvolvME to maintain a close understanding of current health practices and challenges with the focus on the patient-clients' health needs.

CONTRIBUTORS

DOCTOR NATALIE LUSCOMBE-MARSH

Dr Natalie Luscombe-Marsh is a Senior Research Scientist at CSIRO – Health and Biosecurity. She has a PhD in nutrition and disease and expertise in designing clinical and community-based trials in accordance with International Conference on Harmonisation Good Clinical Practice guidelines. Dr Luscombe-Marsh also has expertise in conducting high-quality systematic reviews to provide evidence for general level health claims on food packaging. Her collective research has contributed substantially to knowledge about the effects of foods/dietary patterns, particularly those high in protein and low in carbohydrate on outcomes including appetite, body composition, physical function, hospitalisations, cardio-metabolic risk and quality of life, in young and older adults. Dr Luscombe-Marsh has authored more than 63 peer-reviewed papers and three book chapters, and has received several awards in recognition of the novelty and impact of her work. She is passionate about contributing her expertise to assist industries to innovate and is a voluntary board member of Meals on Wheels South Australia.

PROFESSOR CAMPBELL THOMPSON

Professor Campbell Thompson heads the Acute Medicine Unit at the Royal Adelaide Hospital where he also works in the outpatients department as a senior consultant managing patients with obesity and diabetes. He trained in Sydney and Oxford in the areas of kidney medicine and general medicine and has over 30 years' experience performing clinical metabolic research examining fat deposition and muscle metabolism in health and disease. Currently working at the University of Adelaide, he has published over 200 research articles and supervised over 20 PhD and masters students in the areas of nutrition and metabolism.

DOCTOR TOM WYCHERLEY

Dr Tom Wycherley is a senior lecturer in exercise science at the University of South Australia in Adelaide. Dr Wycherley is an Accredited Exercise Scientist, holds a PhD in nutrition and a master's degree in epidemiology. Tom has over 10 years' experience in evaluating the effects of diet and exercise based programs on weight loss and cardio-metabolic disease risk factors. He has authored more than 40 academic manuscripts on nutrition, physical activity and cardio-metabolic health.

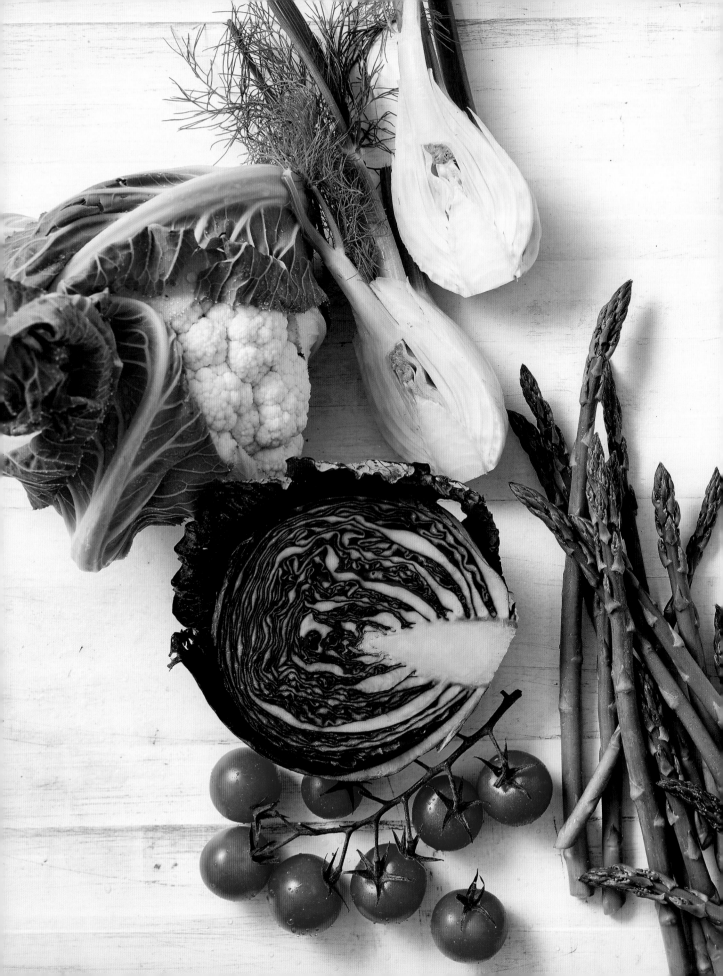

Introduction

FOR MORE THAN 20 YEARS, THE CSIRO HAS BEEN CONDUCTING RESEARCH INTO UNDERSTANDING THE ROLE OF NUTRITIONAL FACTORS AND THE EFFECTS OF HIGHER-PROTEIN, LOWER-CARBOHYDRATE DIETARY APPROACHES FOR WEIGHT AND HEALTH MANAGEMENT, INCLUDING TYPE 2 DIABETES.

This high-quality research continues to challenge and inform clinical nutritional guidelines for managing type 2 diabetes. Between 2012 and 2014, the CSIRO conducted a decisive research study funded by Australia's national governing health body, the National Health and Medical Research Council of Australia (NHMRC), into the effects of a low-carb diet, the results of which have had extremely positive implications for people living with type 2 diabetes. Participants who adopted a low-carb diet – representing an energy-controlled, nutritionally complete eating plan, lower in carbohydrate with higher proportions of protein and healthy fats – combined with a tailored exercise program, were able to reduce their reliance on diabetes medication by an average of 40 per cent, substantially improve their blood sugar control, and achieve significant weight loss. Furthermore, the low-carb diet achieved greater blood glucose control, diabetes medication reduction and improvements in heart health, compared with the traditionally recommended higher-carbohydrate (unrefined), moderate-protein, low-fat diet.

This low-carb diet and lifestyle approach has since been published as **The CSIRO Low-carb Diet**, in a series of three books, all of them bestsellers.

Now, the CSIRO has adapted this popular diet and eating plan in a book specifically for individuals at risk of or living with type 2 diabetes. This already represents so many in society today and continues to grow rapidly. *The CSIRO Low-carb Diabetes Diet & Lifestyle Solution* is a plan designed to help individuals with pre-diabetes and type 2 diabetes understand the condition, and take practical steps to comprehensively improve their health and wellbeing through a complete diet and exercise solution that has been scientifically developed and proven.

Why do we need to worry
ABOUT TYPE 2 DIABETES?

Type 2 diabetes is a progressive disease that affects the body's ability to metabolise glucose (sugar) and maintain optimal blood sugar levels. Without appropriately controlling blood sugar levels and managing symptoms, including through diet and exercise, type 2 diabetes will gradually promote a series of health complications in the individual, including heart disease, high blood pressure, failing eyesight, poor circulation resulting in increased risk of infection and damage to vital body organs. Type 2 diabetes has also been closely linked to the development of dementia and Alzheimer's disease, which is also on the rise in Australia. In addition to having to endure the worry and discomfort of multiple symptoms, individuals with type 2 diabetes often need multiple time-consuming and costly health interventions. This can include medications that may have many negative side-effects and do not necessarily provide the long-term solution. Consequently, individuals with type 2 diabetes might find their enjoyment of life impeded in numerous ways.

At a societal level, the dramatic increase in people affected by type 2 diabetes is linked to the rise in our consumption of highly processed foods and the commensurate jump in our obesity levels. Around 1.7 million Australians have diabetes, many of whom are undiagnosed and unaware of their condition, with many more regarded as having pre-diabetes. Because of the diversity and nature of the symptoms, the cost to the community of caring for individuals with type 2 diabetes is enormous.

We hope this book will make a difference to how Australians understand, prevent and manage type 2 diabetes.

Why is this the right way
TO DEAL WITH TYPE 2 DIABETES?

While many factors contribute to the development of type 2 diabetes – such as age, gender and family history – lifestyle factors are fundamental drivers. What we eat and drink, whether we smoke, whether we exercise and how much sedentary time we spend in our daily lives – these all play a major part in determining our vulnerability to the disease. The positive side of this is that these factors are firmly within our control. That said, we often don't act to improve our health because we don't know what to do. One of the biggest hurdles to developing new habits is the confusion generated by the sheer amount and variability of the information available.

Very few diet products – from books to seminars to online programs – are based on high-quality science. In this environment, it becomes difficult for many of us to know what information to trust and adopt. In contrast, the CSIRO Low-carb Diet was tested rigorously in the 2012–14 randomised controlled trial, and the findings have been supported by more than 20 years of research by other CSIRO studies and research from leading institutions around the world.

THE DIET *in practice*

The CSIRO Low-carb Diabetes Diet & Lifestyle Solution is an energy-controlled, nutritionally complete eating plan based on eating whole, nutrient-dense core foods that provides 50–70 grams of high-quality carbohydrate a day, with proportionally balanced amounts of protein and healthy fats to meet your individual needs. This amount of carbohydrate is equivalent to 3–4 pieces of bread, about 1 cup of rice, or 2 cups of fresh fruit salad. In Australia, we have grown used to consuming much higher levels of carbohydrate, as a result of the increasingly processed nature of discretionary foods in our diet, which typically features bread, rice, pizza, pasta, burgers, pastries, biscuits, desserts and sugary drinks – inexpensive foods, easily prepared, that often include high amounts of added sugars.

As with any changes to your lifestyle, implementing the low-carb diet for daily use can be challenging initially, although many users have reported adapting quickly to the eating plan, not least because they start to see and enjoy benefits quite quickly, such as increased energy and wellbeing, improved sleep and mood, weight loss and – importantly for those with type 2 diabetes – improved blood sugar control with reductions in reliance on medication.

What's in THE BOOK?

When people are well informed about their health and how to take control, their motivation to make improvements increases. To this end, *The CSIRO Low-carb Diabetes Diet & Lifestyle Solution* provides detailed information about type 2 diabetes. It explains the risks and how the disease develops, how it impacts our health, how it is treated and monitored by healthcare professionals, and the vital role of diet and exercise in its management. As above, all the information in the book is based on rigorous CSIRO clinical trials and backed by research from around the world. The practical component of the book contains detailed information with an easy-to-use self-help guide on how to implement the diet and exercise program in your lifestyle. There are visual guides of ingredients to give readers a sense of which foods are high or low in carbs, protein and healthy fats. The twelve weekly meal plans will give those new to the program a clear sense of how the diet works across the day, while 80 recipes show how the diet works, meal by meal. As well, the fully photographed exercise plan provides step-by-step instruction, showing you how to gain full benefit from the low-carb diet.

We hope this book will make a difference to how Australians understand, prevent and manage type 2 diabetes. It is natural to experience the diagnosis of any disease as a major life-setback. It is our hope that the information contained here will help and inspire individuals with type 2 diabetes, and those diagnosed with pre-diabetes, to make the kind of lifestyle changes that can promote dramatic improvements in health and overall enjoyment of life.

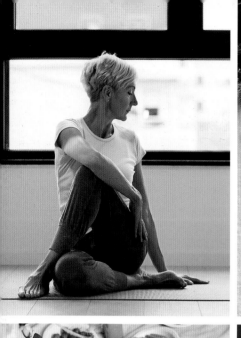
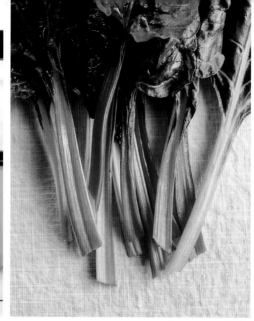
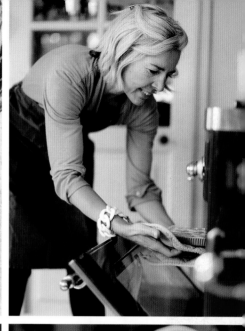
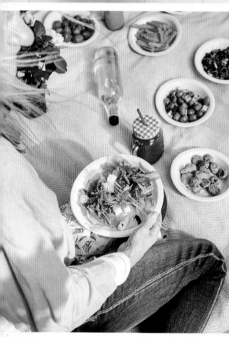

PART

1

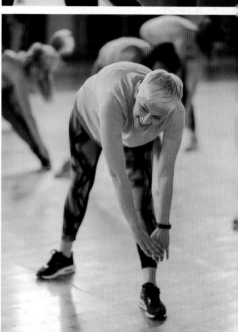
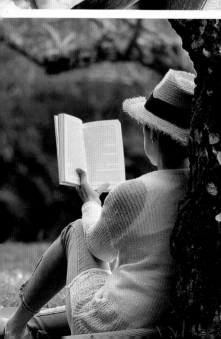
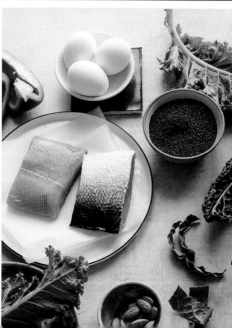
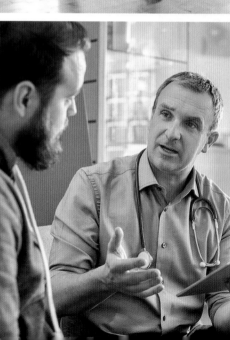

TYPE 2 DIABETES:

A 21st Century Epidemic

Type 2 Diabetes: A 21st Century Epidemic

Diabetes in Australia

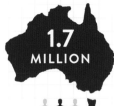

adults living with diabetes

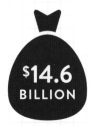

annual cost impact

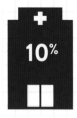

of all hospital admissions are associated with diabetes

TYPE 2 DIABETES HAS BECOME ONE OF THE GREATEST GLOBAL HEALTH CHALLENGES OF THE 21ST CENTURY.

Worldwide, an estimated 415 million individuals are living with diabetes, with 85–90 per cent of cases attributed to type 2 diabetes. By 2045, around 600 million of us may be living with type 2 diabetes. In Australia, an estimated 1.7 million people have diabetes – with an estimated 500,000 said to be undiagnosed type 2 diabetes.

The lifetime risk of developing type 2 diabetes is at least one in three; this means that every third person is likely to develop type 2 diabetes during their life. This risk is not something that starts in older age – many people mistakenly believe type 2 diabetes only affects older people. In fact, it can start affecting people in their 20s and 30s.

The high blood glucose (sugar) levels with diabetes can leave us feeling physically and mentally debilitated, even exhausted and depressed. Poorly controlled diabetes can set you up for poorer health long term, including heart, kidney and eye diseases, and even cancer.

In 2014–15, approximately 10 per cent of all hospital admissions and one in 10 deaths in Australia were associated with diabetes, with type 2 diabetes accounting for over half of all deaths associated with diabetes. Diabetes is estimated to cost the Australian healthcare system $14.6 billion per year – a cost to the individual and to society that is simply not sustainable. With the incidence of type 2 diabetes expected to rise rapidly worldwide, we all have a part to play in reversing this alarming trend.

By reducing your risk of type 2 diabetes and achieving good blood glucose control if you are living with the disease, you will feel so much better and empowered to work towards your life goals.

WHAT IS *type 2 diabetes?*

Type 2 diabetes is a common disease, which is so often talked about that it can be easy to become complacent about its very real health risks. Perhaps you are living with it yourself, or you know of a family member or friend with type 2 diabetes. Increasing numbers of children and adolescents are also being diagnosed. A progressive condition that is often associated with several health complications, including heart disease, type 2 diabetes is also closely linked with high blood pressure and blood cholesterol levels, and even impaired mental health conditions such as depression, dementia and Alzheimer's disease. Thankfully, with some effort and knowledge, type 2 diabetes is a condition that once diagnosed can largely be improved (often without drugs) – and in some cases reversed – through changes to diet and lifestyle.

Formerly known as 'adult onset diabetes' or 'non-insulin dependent diabetes', type 2 diabetes affects the body's ability to metabolise or use glucose (a sugar that is an important metabolic fuel for the body) in cells, resulting in impaired glucose metabolism. With type 2 diabetes, your body either does not produce enough insulin, or it resists the efforts of insulin to properly control blood glucose levels. Insulin is a hormone secreted by the pancreas that allows the body to maintain normal blood glucose (sugar) levels, among other functions.

After eating a meal, blood glucose levels will rise, particularly if that meal is rich in sugars or carbohydrate-rich foods (see page 47) that digest down into glucose (sugar). In response, insulin is released from the pancreas, which causes glucose to move from our bloodstream to our muscles and liver, where it is stored for later use. When glucose metabolism is disrupted and our insulin isn't able to efficiently move the glucose from our blood, the glucose level in our blood increases and remains elevated. This can lead to a state of 'pre-diabetes', a condition that can be present for years before full-blown type 2 diabetes occurs, which is why it is best to start a lifestyle change now – this can prevent type 2 diabetes from developing.

> **With type 2 diabetes, your body either does not produce enough insulin, or it resists the efforts of insulin to properly control blood glucose levels.**

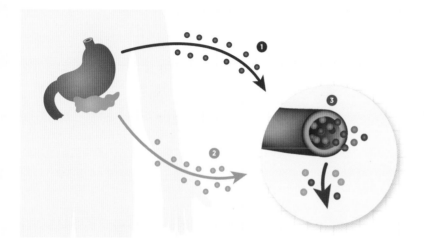

Type 2 diabetes

1. Glucose (sugar) is absorbed into the blood from digested food in the stomach.
2. Insulin is produced in the pancreas and released into the blood.
3. Organs and muscles are less responsive to insulin (insulin resistance) and take up less glucose. Blood sugar levels increase due to insulin resistance.

THE HEALTH CONSEQUENCES
of type 2 diabetes

A person with type 2 diabetes may experience fluctuating blood glucose levels throughout the day and/or night. As they eat – particularly if they eat large amounts of carbohydrate-rich foods – their blood glucose levels rise sharply and to a much higher level ('hyperglycaemia') than in someone who doesn't have diabetes; this is often followed by sharp and dramatic falls in blood glucose. It is these high and fluctuating blood glucose levels that cause many of the health concerns and complications associated with type 2 diabetes, because they damage the blood vessels throughout the body, the heart muscle, eyes and kidneys. Diabetes also changes cell functions, so that cells replicate more rapidly, which explains the association between diabetes and higher rates of some cancers. All these effects can be stopped, and even reversed, with effective timely intervention.

Diabetes complications are varied, and can be grouped into two main categories: **macrovascular diseases,** which affect the large blood vessels to the organs and limbs – adults with type 2 diabetes have a two- to three-fold increased risk of heart attacks and strokes, which account for over half the deaths related to type 2 diabetes; and **microvascular diseases**, which affect the small blood vessels, causing poor circulation within the organs and limbs, and leading to eye disease, kidney failure, poor brain function and nerve damage.

While the effects of type 2 diabetes on physical health are well documented, what many people do not appreciate is its damaging effects on mental health and performance. It is well established that type 2 diabetes increases the risk of depression and anxiety. Scientific evidence increasingly shows that chronic exposure to high blood glucose levels can decrease cognitive function and is also closely linked to the development of dementia and Alzheimer's disease. (Some researchers have described this as 'type 3 diabetes'.) Once dementia is diagnosed and pathological changes become evident, it is difficult to reverse its progression.

With the prevalence of Alzheimer's disease and dementia increasing in Australia, this should be reason enough to take action now to improve and optimise your blood glucose control and reduce your risk of type 2 diabetes, so that you can maintain the health of your brain and its daily functioning throughout your entire life.

Just to summarise: diabetes is a major cause of blindness, kidney failure, heart attacks, stroke and lower limb amputation. Type 2 diabetes also increases the risk of mental health disorders including depression, cognitive impairment, dementia and Alzheimer's disease.

Remember, it is the constantly high and widely fluctuating blood glucose levels that cause the health complications associated with type 2 diabetes. This is why controlling blood glucose levels is the primary target. Using strategies that will both lower blood glucose levels and promote a more stable blood glucose profile across the day will help reduce these health risks.

> It is the constantly high and widely fluctuating blood glucose levels that cause the health complications associated with type 2 diabetes.

THE DAMAGE DIABETES CAN DO

General
High blood glucose
Low blood glucose
Widely fluctuating blood glucose
High blood cholesterol
Emotional distress and isolation
Higher rates of cancer such as colon, breast,
endometrial (uterine) and pancreas

Brain
Increased stroke risk
Cognitive impairment
Depression
Increased risk of dementia and Alzheimer's

Eyes
Cataracts
Damage to retina
Nerve damage

Heart
Faster hardening of the arteries
Heart attack
Irregular heartbeat

Blood pressure effects
Dizziness on standing
High blood pressure

Stomach and intestines
Delayed stomach emptying
Diarrhoea

Kidneys
Kidney disease or damage
Urinary tract infections

Poor wound healing

Genital and urinary
Fertility issues
Bladder not emptying
Urinary tract infections

Skin
Fungal infections
Bacterial infections
Diabetic rash
Areas of increased pigmentation
Areas of pigmentation loss

Muscle wasting

Blood vessels in the extremities
Macrovascular (large blood vessel) disease
Microvascular (small blood vessel) disease

Peripheral nerve damage
Pins and needles
Muscle weakness
Reduced reflexes
Pain and/or numbness

Foot problems
Pain at rest
Ulcers
Gangrene (leading to amputation)

How does TYPE 2 DIABETES DEVELOP?

Developing diabetes is a matter of whether you have the underlying genes, but the genes are very common – consider the high diabetes rates and think about your own family history. To understand how type 2 diabetes develops, it is important to know that when we eat, our digestive process turns any carbohydrate in our food into glucose, which is released into the bloodstream and taken up by the cells in our body to be stored or used as fuel. When we eat carbohydrate-rich foods, this conversion process can be very rapid, and leads to a sudden rise in the level of glucose in our blood.

In response to this blood glucose spike, the pancreas (an organ next to the stomach) produces insulin, a hormone that allows cells throughout the body to take up and use the glucose as fuel, or to store it for later (in fat, muscle or the liver), to maintain a normal blood glucose level.

In a normal state of blood glucose control, the pancreas and the liver interact in a tightly controlled system to regulate the release and action of insulin. However, over time, due to a number of contributing factors – some genetic, but mostly lifestyle-related, including insufficient physical activity, excessive energy intake and obesity – a state of insulin resistance can develop, whereby cells become less responsive to the insulin signal, meaning that insulin becomes increasingly ineffective and glucose no longer efficiently moves into cells.

Insulin resistance makes it difficult for our body to control our blood glucose, causing our blood glucose levels to remain high. As our body becomes more resistant to the action of insulin and it is less able to move glucose into cells, the pancreas starts to produce greater amounts of insulin, which can lead to high blood insulin levels ('hyperinsulinaemia'). This reduced capacity to maintain normal blood glucose levels then starts to lead to high blood glucose levels ('hyperglycaemia'), which results in a state of **glucose intolerance** or **pre-diabetes**, where our glucose levels remain above the normal range.

This higher level of insulin also promotes body fat storage, and it comes to a point where the fat cells become so enlarged and inflamed that they can no longer hold any more, so fat starts to accumulate around the vital organs such as the liver, pancreas and heart, which is termed visceral fat. It is the visceral fat that is much worse for your health than the fat around your thighs and buttocks.

In some cases, if left untreated, this constant need to produce more and more insulin can put so much stress on the pancreas that it begins to wear out, and its ability to produce and release insulin declines. Around the time someone is diagnosed with type 2 diabetes, they have lost 50–70 per cent of their functional insulin-producing cells.

> Insulin resistance makes it difficult for our body to control our blood glucose, causing our blood glucose levels to remain high.

Ultimately, this means the body is left in a permanent state of hyperglycaemia. The body will remain in this state unless the diet is changed to deliver less glucose or a blood glucose-controlling medication such as metformin or insulin is used. Think of the pancreas as being similar to a car engine: if overworked, it will burn out and stop working, meaning an external power source will be needed to get things moving again.

This shows why undertaking early effective treatment strategies that improve blood glucose control and reduce blood glucose levels are so important in preventing and managing type 2 diabetes. Such strategies include lifestyle changes that promote a healthy weight and increased physical activity levels, which can be of great benefit in improving insulin sensitivity and reducing blood glucose levels.

THE PROGRESSION OF TYPE 2 DIABETES

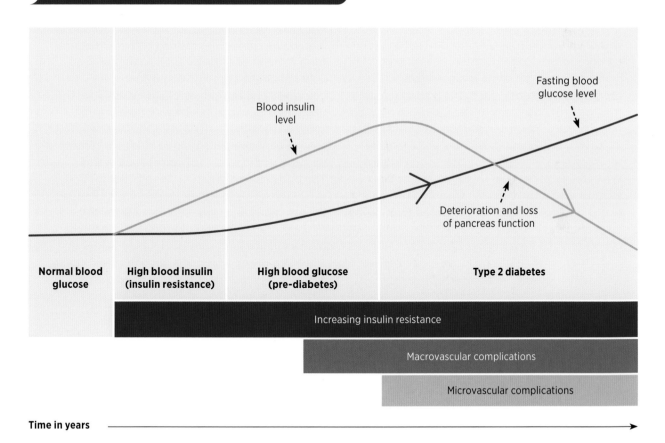

What happens when I eat carbohydrate-containing foods?

Carbohydrate digestion is the process by which our body converts carbohydrate-containing foods – such as bread, cereals, rice, pasta, potatoes, milk, fruit, sugar-sweetened beverages, honey and table sugar (see 'Where do I find carbohydrates?' on page 47) – into simple forms of sugar, such as glucose, to provide fuel (energy) for our body.

The mechanical breakdown of carbohydrates begins in the mouth, as we chew food into pieces. Chewing also stimulates the release of a salivary enzyme called amylase, which breaks carbohydrates into smaller forms of sugars, to be transported to the gut for further digestion.

After the carbohydrate is digested in the gut, the glucose is absorbed into the bloodstream, triggering the pancreas to release insulin into the bloodstream. Insulin is a hormone that is needed to move glucose into the muscle and liver cells for storage as glycogen, for later use as energy. While the liver can hold up to 100 grams of glucose, and muscle tissue can store 400–500 grams of glucose (in its concentrated form called glycogen), excess glucose beyond the glycogen capacity of the liver and muscle tissue is converted to fat (triglyceride; see page 28) and moved into fat cells for longer-term storage.

By the time type 2 diabetes is present, the muscle and liver cells have become less responsive to insulin ('insulin resistant'), and/or the pancreas cannot produce enough insulin to help pull the glucose out of the blood for storage. As a result, instead of being stored for later energy needs, the glucose in the blood rises to higher levels. If uncontrolled, prolonged high blood glucose levels lead to further declines in pancreas function, to the point where medications become necessary for diabetes management.

Exceptions

The most notable exception to the carbohydrate metabolism process explained above is **dietary fibre** (contained in foods such as wholegrains, vegetables and legumes including lentils, chickpeas and red kidney beans, which also contain carbohydrates). Dietary fibre is a carbohydrate that can be classed as either soluble (dissolves in water) or insoluble (cannot be dissolved in water), or as resistant starch. The body cannot digest or absorb dietary fibre in the same way as other carbohydrates. Instead, these indigestible carbohydrates are partially broken down (fermented) in the large intestine by bacteria to form short-chain fatty acids, which are needed for good gut and bowel health. Indigestible fibres pass through the digestive system and are removed when you empty your bowel.

How is TYPE 2 DIABETES DIAGNOSED?

GPs can diagnose **pre-diabetes** ('a higher than normal blood glucose level') and **diabetes** relatively easily by measuring blood glucose levels and comparing them to the values in the table below. Separate blood samples can be taken first thing in the morning before eating ('fasting blood glucose'), and after drinking a fluid containing a standardised dose (75 grams) of glucose.

Pre-diabetes or diabetes will be diagnosed if your fasting blood glucose levels are high, or if your blood glucose rises higher than a certain level after taking the glucose drink.

Another standard blood test used to diagnose diabetes measures **glycosylated haemoglobin (HbA1c)** – which is a way of describing the average amount of glucose that has become attached to haemoglobin (the oxygen-carrying molecule in your red blood cells) over the past 3 months (which is the lifespan of a red blood cell). This test indicates the average level of glucose in your blood for the past 3 months. If your glucose levels have been high over recent weeks, your HbA1c level will be higher.

DIAGNOSING DIABETES

Condition	Fasting blood glucose (mmol/L)	Blood glucose 2 hours after ingestion of 75 g glucose (mmol/L)*	HbA1c levels	
			(per cent)	(mmol/mol)
Normal	3.9–5.5	less than 7.8	less than 5.7	less than 39
Pre-diabetes	5.6–6.9	7.8–11	5.7–6.4	39–47
Diabetes	7.0 or more	more than 11	6.5 or more	48 or more

Note: HbA1c levels will be given either as a percentage (old unit) or as mmol/mol (new unit). Only one of these is required for a diagnosis of diabetes. *Oral glucose tolerance test

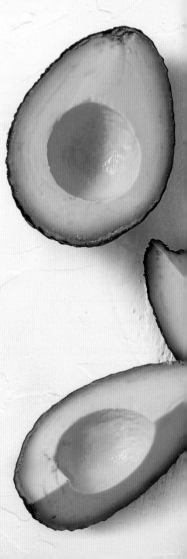

A key reason these tests are used to classify and monitor diabetes status and blood glucose control is that research shows that if these measures can be reduced (indicating that blood glucose control is better), the risk of developing diabetes complications is reduced, or their progression is prevented.

In addition to these standard measures of blood glucose control, emerging research shows that **daily blood glucose variability** – which describes how much your blood glucose level fluctuates up and down across the day, and the size of the swings – is an independent risk factor for diabetes health complications. This means that irrespective of your HbA1c and fasting blood glucose levels, having widely oscillating blood glucose levels across the day is associated with greater risk of health complications and heart disease.

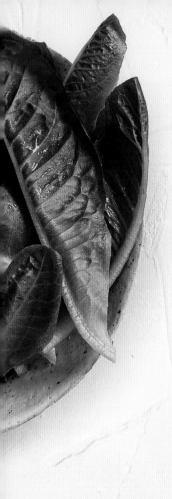

The graph below shows how two people with the same average blood glucose level (HbA1c) can have very different glycaemic (blood glucose) variability levels. **Person 1** has relatively stable blood glucose, while **Person 2** has a blood glucose profile that fluctuates widely throughout the day, putting them at much greater risk of health complications. This is why, when considering treatment options for diabetes management, the best solutions are those that both:

1. reduce fasting blood glucose and HbA1c levels;
2. minimise the post-eating rises in blood glucose, and the level of glucose variability across the day.

Remember!

Treatment options that both lower blood glucose levels **and** stabilise blood glucose patterns across the day are the best way to reduce the health risks associated with diabetes.

SAME HBA1C – VERY DIFFERENT GLYCAEMIC VARIABILITY

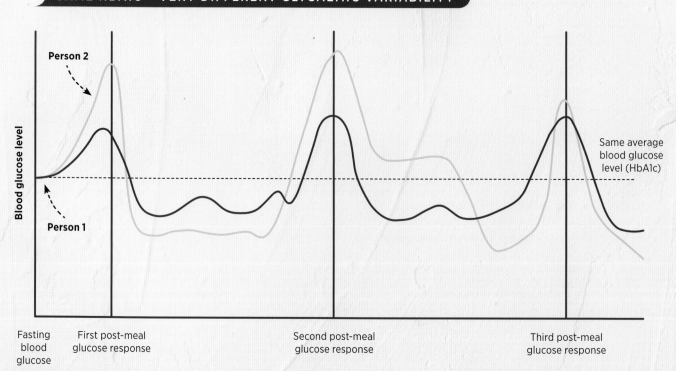

BLOOD GLUCOSE MONITORING
for effective diabetes management

If you have diabetes, it is always a good idea to keep a close check on your blood glucose levels. A simple way to do this at home is with a finger-prick blood test, using a device called a **glucometer** (a glucose meter), together with a lancet (to prick your finger) and glucose test strips (to measure the glucose in your blood). Tests should generally be performed at various times throughout the day: in the morning before breakfast (to check your fasting blood glucose), and 2 hours after lunch and dinner (to check your post-meal glucose), and may be done over a specified period (e.g. four measures daily for 2 weeks). Another option is a **continuous glucose monitoring device** (see page 63), which monitors your blood glucose constantly across the whole day.

Collecting these blood glucose readings can help you and your healthcare team to establish blood glucose targets that are individual to your needs and treatment, such as if medications are needed. If you have type 2 diabetes, it is important that you develop a plan for self-monitoring your blood glucose levels, to determine if you are effectively managing your type 2 diabetes, or if your blood glucose pattern is changing, so that you and your healthcare team can adjust how your diabetes is being managed. Measuring your blood glucose levels gives you the advantage of knowing immediately whether any symptoms you might be experiencing are caused by hypoglycaemia (low blood glucose levels) or hyperglycaemia (high blood glucose levels). This will help you to take corrective lifestyle action to regain blood glucose control.

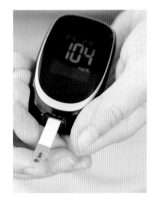

It is important that you develop a plan for self-monitoring your blood glucose levels.

HOW LOW IS TOO LOW?
Hypoglycaemia is defined as having blood glucose levels less than 4.0 mmol/L. It can cause symptoms including:

▶ increased hunger (polyphagia)

▶ increased sweating

▶ poor memory

▶ slurred speech

▶ dizziness and even blackouts.

You are only likely to experience hypoglycaemia if you are taking medication that lowers your blood glucose levels, such as insulin or a sulphonylurea (for example gliclazide, gliclazide ER, glibenclamide, glipizide or glimepiride). If you are on these medications and you choose to change your level of carbohydrate intake (particularly if you are reducing it), it is recommended that you do this under the supervision of an accredited practising dietitian and your GP. This is because having a lower amount of carbohydrate in your diet is likely to cause your blood glucose levels to reduce, meaning you will need less of these medications. Other blood glucose–lowering medications (such as metformin or glitazones; see page 62) do not cause hypoglycaemia. If you are on other medications and feeling as though you are experiencing symptoms, test your blood glucose levels and/or speak to your GP.

Your GP and healthcare team will help you to define your blood glucose level targets.

HOW HIGH IS TOO HIGH?

Hyperglycaemia occurs with blood glucose levels greater than 10 mmol/L. Often, blood glucose levels this high do not have obvious symptoms, but when there are symptoms, these can include:

▶ increased urinary frequency (polyuria)

▶ increased thirst (polydipsia)

▶ fatigue

▶ blurred vision.

SO, WHAT ARE THE RECOMMENDED BLOOD GLUCOSE LEVEL TARGETS?

Effective blood glucose management will achieve levels within the range of **4–8 mmol/L** for **fasting blood glucose**. Your GP and healthcare team will help you to define your targets based on your age, how long you have had diabetes, the type of medical and nutrition treatment regime you are following, and your physical activity levels.

If you are measuring your blood glucose levels at home, Diabetes Australia suggests the following targets:

TARGET LEVELS AT HOME (NON-FASTING)

Timing of test	mmol/L
Before meals	4–8
2 hours after the start of a meal	6–10

If you have well-controlled diabetes, you should have your GP check your HbA1c every 6 months. If you are newly diagnosed or have unstable diabetes (difficulty reaching stable glucose levels), a GP check every 3 months may be more suitable until good control is established. An **HbA1c of 6.5–7 per cent (48–53 mmol/mol)** is considered to indicate good control.

While it is important to self-monitor your blood glucose levels to ensure they stay as close to these target ranges as possible, to reduce your risk of developing complications, it is also important that you check your levels with your GP or a credentialled diabetes educator (CDE) to help you manage any changes in glucose control that may arise.

If you do not have type 2 diabetes and wish to use a glucometer to measure your blood glucose levels to identify how your body responds to foods, it is advisable that you speak to your local pharmacist, who can help you to select a suitable glucometer and provide advice on how to use it.

RISK FACTORS *for type 2 diabetes*

So far we have looked at the health consequences of type 2 diabetes, how the condition develops, and how it is diagnosed. Let's now take a closer look at the general lifestyle and genetic factors that make a person more likely to develop the disease, and what can be done to address these. Research tells us there are several important non-modifiable and modifiable risk factors associated with pre-diabetes and type 2 diabetes.

NON-MODIFIABLE RISK FACTORS

Non-modifiable risk factors are those that cannot be changed in any way, by either lifestyle choices or medications. For type 2 diabetes, these include:

- **advancing age**
- **sex** (with men having greater risk)
- **a family history** of diabetes (a mother, father or sibling with diabetes)
- **ethnicity** (with people having an Aboriginal, Torres Strait Islander, Middle Eastern, Asian, Pacific Island, Indian Subcontinent, African American, Latino or Native American background being at greater risk).

MODIFIABLE RISK FACTORS

Modifiable risk factors are those that can be changed, whether by diet and lifestyle choices or medications. For type 2 diabetes, these include:

- **obesity and abdominal obesity**, especially abdominal or visceral obesity (the excess body fat stored in the abdominal region and around vital organs)
- **an abnormal blood cholesterol (fat) profile**, with high levels of unhealthy cholesterol – triglycerides and LDL (low-density lipoprotein) cholesterol – and/or low levels of good cholesterol – HDL (high-density lipoprotein) cholesterol
- **high blood pressure**
- **elevated blood glucose levels**.

This cluster of conditions – abdominal obesity, abnormal blood cholesterol profile, high blood pressure and elevated blood glucose levels – has been shown to substantially increase the risk of type 2 diabetes. See page 26 for more on this. Further important and far more easily modifiable risk factors for type 2 diabetes include an unhealthy diet, lack of physical activity and high levels of sedentary time, alcohol intake and tobacco smoking.

This is why strategies that can reduce and reverse these modifiable risk factors are so vitally important to decrease your risk and delay the onset of type 2 diabetes.

Risk factors for type 2 diabetes

NON-MODIFIABLE

Advancing age

Sex (male)

Ethnicity

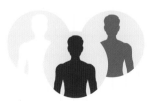

Family history

MODIFIABLE

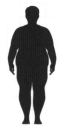

Obesity and
abdominal obesity

Abnormal blood
cholesterol levels

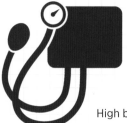

High blood
pressure

Elevated blood
glucose levels

Poor diet

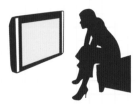

Physical inactivity
and high levels of
sedentary time

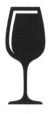

Alcohol

Tobacco smoking

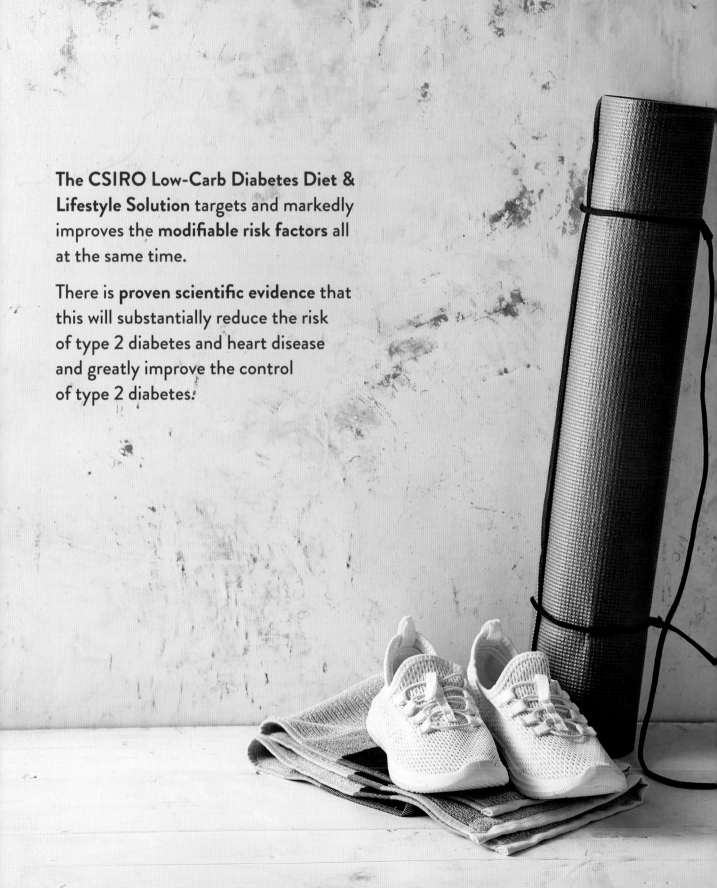

The CSIRO Low-Carb Diabetes Diet & Lifestyle Solution targets and markedly improves the modifiable risk factors all at the same time.

There is proven scientific evidence that this will substantially reduce the risk of type 2 diabetes and heart disease and greatly improve the control of type 2 diabetes.

A closer look at the
MODIFIABLE RISK FACTORS

There are four important modifiable risk factors: abdominal obesity, abnormal blood fat levels, high blood pressure, and elevated blood glucose levels.

OBESITY

About 80–85 per cent of people with type 2 diabetes are also overweight or obese. Given the rising global obesity rates, which have nearly tripled since 1975 to epidemic levels, with more than 1.9 billion adults now overweight and over 650 million obese, it is not surprising that an explosion in type 2 diabetes has occurred. To determine whether you are overweight or obese, calculate your **body mass index (BMI)** using the equation below and then compare it with the values in the table opposite. If you would prefer to use an online tool to calculate your BMI, visit **healthyweight.health.gov.au/ wps/portal/Home/helping-hand/bmi.**

Waist circumference is another useful measure for obtaining an estimate of your risk of developing a long-term disease. As a general rule, the waist measurement should be no more than 88 cm for women and no more than 102 cm for men – greater than this indicates the presence of excess abdominal fat. You can use your BMI in combination with your waist circumference to determine your risk of conditions such as insulin resistance, type 2 diabetes and heart disease (see opposite).

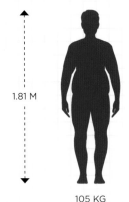

1.81 M

105 KG

Sample BMI calculation

Gary is 181 centimetres (i.e. 1.81 metres) tall and weighs 105 kilograms. His BMI is therefore:

$$BMI\ (kg/m^2) = weight\ (kg)\ /\ (height\ (m)\ x\ height\ (m))$$
$$= 105\ /\ (1.81\ x\ 1.81)$$
$$= 32\ (rounded\ down)$$

Comparing this value to those in the table opposite, Gary can see he's in the obese class 1 category and would benefit from losing weight.

How to measure your waist circumference:

❱ Find the top of your hip bone and take the measurement just above this.

❱ Ensure the tape measure is level with your belly button and parallel to the floor.

❱ Don't hold your breath, and take the measurement at the end of a breath out.

❱ Aim to have the tape snug (but not tight) around your waist.

USING BMI AND WAIST CIRCUMFERENCE TO ASSESS METABOLIC DISEASE RISK

Weight classification	BMI (kg/m^2)	Metabolic disease risk	
		Waist circumference less than 88 cm (women)/102 cm (men)	Waist circumference greater than 88 cm (women)/102 cm (men)
Underweight	Less than 18.49	–	–
Healthy (normal)	18.50–24.99	–	–
Overweight (pre-obese)	25.00–29.99	Increased	High
Obese class I	30.00–34.99	High	Very high
Obese class II	35.00–39.99	Very high	Very high
Obese class III	40.00 or more	Extremely high	Extremely high

Source: Adapted from WHO, apps.who.int/bmi/index.jsp?introPage=intro_3.html

There's some debate about the most appropriate cut-offs of BMI and waist circumference measurements for different ethnic groups, including Aboriginal and Torres Strait Islander people, and people of Asian and Pacific heritage. The World Health Organization (WHO) estimates that in different Asian populations the risk of developing type 2 diabetes and heart disease increases with a BMI of 22–25 and a waist circumference of more than 80 centimetres for women and 90 centimetres for men. Whatever your ethnicity, BMI can't take into account your individual body composition – how much body fat or muscle you have – so you should always use your BMI and/or waist circumference only as a guide. If your BMI and metabolic disease risk do come out high, though, start with a visit to your GP as soon as you can for blood glucose tests.

ABNORMAL BLOOD CHOLESTEROL (FAT) LEVELS

Having high levels of unhealthy fats and low levels of healthy fat in your blood can increase the risk of type 2 diabetes and heart disease. Unhealthy fats are triglycerides and low-density lipoprotein (LDL or 'bad' cholesterol) that increase the risk of heart disease, whereas high-density lipoprotein (HDL or 'good' cholesterol) is considered a healthy fat that will reduce heart disease risk. An unhealthy blood fat profile can be influenced by several factors including genetics, poor diet, lack of exercise and smoking.

WHAT ARE BLOOD FATS?

Cholesterol and triglycerides are two forms of blood fats that are necessary for life itself. Both can either be produced within the body or come from dietary sources. The scientific word for fats is lipids, so you may hear your healthcare team talking about your blood lipid levels.

Cholesterol is a white, insoluble, waxy substance produced by the liver and most cells in the body. It's essential for many processes of daily life, including building cell membranes and brain and nerve cells, and producing the bile acids that absorb fats and the fat-soluble vitamins (A, D, E and K). The body also uses cholesterol to make vitamin D and key hormones that help our metabolism work efficiently.

Triglycerides are fats made up of groups of three high-energy fatty acid chains connected by a glycerol molecule. The fatty acids are absorbed from food by the intestine or produced by the liver from glucose. They provide body cells with fuel to function. If unused, triglycerides are stored in either body fat deposits until required or in the liver, sometimes building up to excess levels causing a 'fatty liver' that is now affecting 20 per cent of the developed world. Fatty liver is known to interfere with the function of insulin and is one of the causes of type 2 diabetes itself.

Cholesterol and triglycerides cannot circulate freely in the blood because blood is mostly water. Instead, they're packaged with proteins and other substances to form soluble particles called *lipoproteins*. There are several different types of lipoprotein, each with a different purpose. The two main types of lipoprotein we measure are:

▶ **low-density lipoprotein (LDL) cholesterol.** This delivers cholesterol to cells and is often called 'bad' cholesterol because when levels in the blood are too high, it builds up and sticks to the lining of the blood vessels. This stimulates the formation of plaques within the arteries and leads to atherosclerosis (hardening of the arteries). LDL cholesterol is a particularly important consideration for those with high risk for heart disease, which includes individuals with type 2 diabetes

▶ **high-density lipoprotein (HDL) cholesterol.** This helps remove excess cholesterol from the cells, including arterial cells, and is therefore called 'good' cholesterol.

High levels of unhealthy fats and low levels of healthy fat in your blood can increase the risk of type 2 diabetes and heart disease.

MONITORING BLOOD FATS

A test of blood fat content, often a fasting blood test, can indicate the risk of a heart attack or stroke in the next five years. Treatment that lowers the levels of triglycerides and LDL cholesterol (bad cholesterol) reduces the risk of heart attack, while strategies that elevate levels of HDL cholesterol (good cholesterol) also reduce the risk of heart disease. The great news is that *The CSIRO Low-Carb Diabetes Diet & Lifestyle Solution* does exactly that. It will markedly improve your blood fat profile by reducing your triglyceride and LDL cholesterol levels and increasing your HDL cholesterol levels. This will significantly improve your diabetes control and reduce your risk of heart disease.

BLOOD FATS TARGET

Australian Government guidelines recommend that we have our health, and particularly our heart health, assessed every two years after the age of 45. This includes having our blood glucose and blood fat levels checked. If your levels indicate a borderline–high risk of developing heart disease (see below), it is best to make changes to your diet and exercise habits (aiming for a modest weight reduction of around 5 kg) to help bring your blood fat levels down. If they remain elevated, and you are at high risk of heart disease, you may be prescribed cholesterol-lowering medication, most often statins.

Blood fat (mmol/L)	Low risk	Borderline	High risk
LDL cholesterol	Less than 1.8	More than 2	More than 4.5
HDL cholesterol	At least 1	Less than 1	Less than 0.9
Triglyceride	Less than 2	2 or more	More than 6

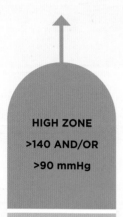

HIGH ZONE
>140 AND/OR
>90 mmHg

NORMAL TO NORMAL-HIGH ZONE
120-139 AND/OR
80-89 mmHg

OPTIMAL ZONE
<120 AND/OR
<80 mmHg

HIGH BLOOD PRESSURE

The higher your blood pressure, the greater your risk of developing type 2 diabetes, and one or more of the following health concerns: heart attack, heart failure, stroke, kidney failure and poor circulation. Effective ways to control blood pressure include a diet low in salt, plenty of exercise, reducing your alcohol intake if you consume alcohol, and, if you're overweight or obese, losing weight. *The CSIRO Low-Carb Diabetes Diet & Lifestyle Solution* will help you achieve all of these. Recent evidence has also highlighted the role of insulin levels and high blood pressure in type 2 diabetes, where insulin causes the kidneys to store salt. Since a lower-carbohydrate diet can cause insulin levels to fall, it promotes the kidneys to release the salt that can potentially reduce blood pressure and even stop the need for blood-pressure lowering medication. However, in some instances, even if you make these lifestyle changes you might also need prescription medication to help keep your blood pressure down. If you have high blood pressure with low levels of physical activity and/or a poor diet, it is highly likely you will need to take medication to help control your blood pressure, so you don't put your body systems (such as your heart, eyes and liver) at greater risk.

MEASURING BLOOD PRESSURE

Blood pressure is usually given with an upper reading (which health practitioners call systolic blood pressure) and a lower reading (diastolic blood pressure), in millimetres of mercury (mmHg). Both readings are important, and adults should generally aim for a blood pressure in the normal to normal–high zone. As you no doubt know, blood pressure is generally measured using an inflatable cuff around the upper arm. Assessing your blood pressure control relies on regular measurements. Portable blood pressure monitors are easy to purchase at a reasonable price, so that you can keep track of your blood pressure at home. This is especially useful if your blood pressure rises steeply when you visit your GP! Blood pressure can vary significantly during the day, so a 24-hour recording from an automated monitor or a diary of readings from a manual monitor, collected under the same conditions each time (e.g. after sitting quietly at a table for 5 minutes), can help your healthcare team understand your blood pressure control over time. This is especially important if you're losing weight, as blood pressure usually falls as weight is lost. An automated monitor can also identify people whose blood pressure doesn't fall while they sleep, a condition that requires particular treatment.

BLOOD PRESSURE TARGETS

You and your healthcare team should discuss an acceptable blood pressure target for you, but usually this will be around 120/80 mmHg (or a little higher in people over 70). If you have proteinuria (protein in the urine, an indicator of kidney damage), you may even be given a lower blood pressure target than this. A treatment is working if your blood pressure drops – simple as that. This indicates good health outcomes, such as lower levels of protein in the urine and a reduction in the thickness of the heart muscle (which, if necessary, can be checked using an ultrasound of the heart). For older people, however, a lower blood pressure target may not be appropriate. This is because low blood pressure can increase the risk of a fall.

MONITORING BLOOD PRESSURE

If you're taking blood pressure medication and at the same time losing weight thanks to lifestyle modifications, your healthcare team will need to monitor your blood pressure levels closely. This is necessary to prevent it falling too low, which can cause faintness or dizziness. If your blood pressure falls and you're still losing weight or maintaining a lower weight, your medication dose may need to be adjusted or stopped altogether. Since blood pressure medications can have side effects, reducing or stopping medication not only saves you money but may further improve your health and wellbeing.

If despite making lifestyle changes your blood pressure is still not fully under control, you may need antihypertensive (blood-pressure lowering) medication prescribed by your GP.

ELEVATED BLOOD GLUCOSE LEVELS

Having elevated blood glucose levels above the normal range significantly increases your risk of developing type 2 diabetes, and will classify you as having a pre-diabetes status. Elevated blood glucose levels mean that the body is already showing early signs that it is starting to struggle to effectively metabolise and remove glucose from the blood, which if left untreated over the long term can result in a range of health consequences (see page 14).

Measuring and monitoring blood glucose levels can be easily achieved with a home-based finger-prick blood test, using a glucometer, lancet and glucose test strip as described on page 21.

Are you at risk of type 2 diabetes?

A delay in diagnosing type 2 diabetes is often a result of the symptoms not being severe enough to be recognised, compounded by the fact that the symptoms develop slowly over time.

This is why it is always a good idea to have annual checks with your GP who can test whether you have diabetes and/or the risk factors.

If you would like to determine your risk of developing type 2 diabetes in the next 5 years, you can complete the risk assessment over the page (or visit baker.edu.au/health-hub/diabetes-risk-assessment).

DIABETES RISK ASSESSMENT

1 **What is your age group?**

Under 35	0 points
35–44	2 points
45–54	4 points
55–64	6 points
65 or over	8 points

2 **What is your gender?**

Female	0 points
Male	3 points

3 **What are your ethnicity and your country of birth?**

Are you of Aboriginal, Torres Strait Islander, Pacific Islander or Maori descent?

No	0 points
Yes	2 points

Where were you born?

Australia	0 points
Asia	2 points
Indian subcontinent	2 points
Middle East	2 points
North Africa	2 points
Southern Europe	2 points
Other	0 points

4 **Have either of your parents, or any of your brothers or sisters been diagnosed with diabetes (type 1 or type 2)?**

No	0 points
Yes	3 points

5 **Have you ever been found to have high blood glucose (sugar) in a health examination, during an illness or during pregnancy?**

No	0 points
Yes	6 points

6 **Are you currently taking medication for high blood pressure?**

No	0 points
Yes	2 points

7 **Do you currently smoke cigarettes or any other tobacco products on a daily basis?**

No	0 points
Yes	2 points

8 How often do you eat vegetables or fruit?

Every day	0 points
Not every day	1 point

9 On average, would you say you do at least 2.5 hours of physical activity per week (for example, 30 minutes a day on five or more days a week)?

Yes	0 points
No	2 points

10 What is your waist measurement taken below the ribs (usually at the level of the navel, and while standing)?

For those of Asian, Aboriginal or Torres Strait Islander descent

Men	Women	
▶ Less than 90 cm	Less than 80 cm	0 points
▶ 90–100 cm	80–90 cm	4 points
▶ More than 100 cm	More than 90 cm	7 points

For all others

Men	Women	
▶ Less than 102 cm	Less than 88 cm	0 points
▶ 102–110 cm	88–100 cm	4 points
▶ More than 110 cm	More than 100 cm	7 points

YOUR RISK OF DEVELOPING TYPE 2 DIABETES WITHIN 5 YEARS

Check your total score against the three point ranges below. Note that if you're less than 25 years old, the overall score may overestimate your risk of diabetes.

5 OR LESS: LOW RISK
Approximately one person in every 100 with a score in this range will develop diabetes.

6–11: INTERMEDIATE RISK
Approximately one person in every 50 with a score in the range of 6–8 will develop diabetes. Approximately one person in every 30 with a score in the range of 9–11 will develop diabetes. Discuss your score with your GP and consider lifestyle changes to reduce your risk.

12 OR MORE: HIGH RISK
Approximately one person in every 14 with a score in the range of 12–15 will develop diabetes. Approximately one person in every seven with a score in the range of 16–19 will develop diabetes. Approximately one person in every three with a score in the range of 20 and above will develop diabetes. You may have undiagnosed diabetes. See your GP as soon as possible for a fasting glucose test.

Now for the GOOD NEWS

If you have been diagnosed with pre-diabetes or type 2 diabetes, or you have any of the modifiable risk factors for type 2 diabetes, or you simply just need to lose some weight, the good news is that there is help at hand. These are all targets that can be easily improved, all at the same time, by the eating and exercise plan provided in this book.

What's more, it is a scientifically proven solution that can reduce all of these modifiable risk factors, improve the management of type 2 diabetes, and also improve your overall wellbeing, making you feel great and allowing you to live that active, healthy life that you deserve. Even more, in some cases you can achieve these benefits while also reducing or even eliminating some or all of your medications, which means less cost – and more importantly, fewer side effects and better health.

All these health targets can be easily improved, all at the same time, by the eating and exercise plan provided in this book.

These targets and health improvements include:

- reducing your weight and waist circumference (abdominal obesity)
- lowering your blood pressure
- improving your blood fat profile (by decreasing your triglycerides and LDL cholesterol levels, and increasing your HDL cholesterol levels)
- better controlling your blood glucose levels – which includes reducing your fasting blood glucose levels, HbA1c, post-meal spikes and blood glucose fluctuations throughout the day (the degree to which your blood glucose levels go up and down, also known as glycaemic variability)
- increasing your physical activity level
- improving your overall diet quality.

In fact, the changes listed above are also the same key factors that your GP will focus on in improving your health and wellbeing. So by simply making the changes outlined in this book, you can reduce all of these risk factors, in addition to gaining many other benefits, providing you with a complete wellness solution. Some people who have tried this approach have reported how amazed their GPs have been by the changes they have been able to achieve.

Research also shows that the development and progression of diabetes-related health complications are primarily related to the duration and magnitude of these modifiable risk factors. So acting now and gaining all the benefits of this plan today will help you live a longer, higher-quality life.

Importantly, undertaking this plan in close consultation and collaboration with your GP and healthcare team can help you tailor this plan to your own personal needs and preferences, and integrate it within your pre-existing medical management plan.

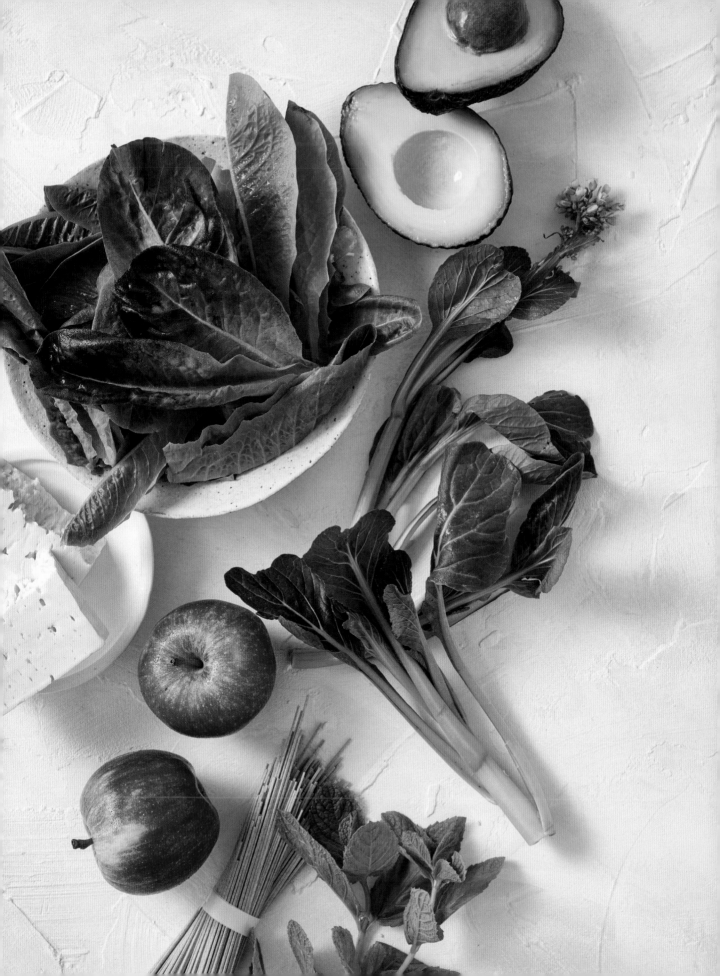

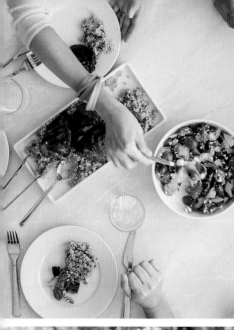
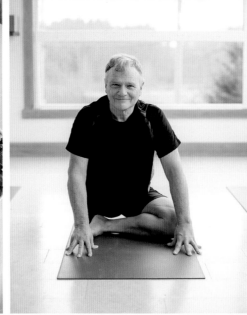
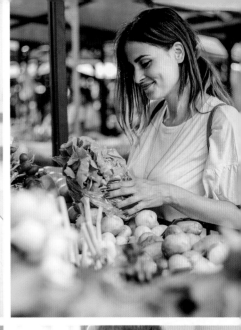
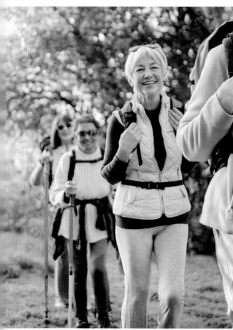

PART

2

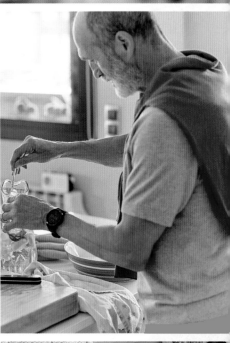
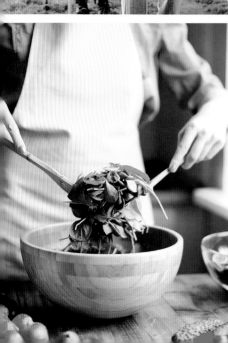
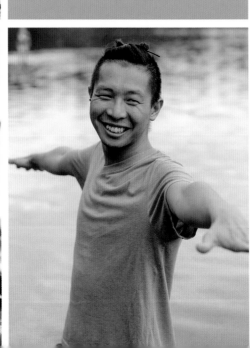
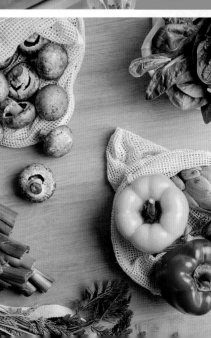

THE CSIRO LOW-CARB DIABETES

diet & lifestyle solution

The CSIRO Low-carb Diabetes Diet & Lifestyle Solution

THE FIRST-LINE TREATMENT FOR MANAGING OBESITY AND TYPE 2 DIABETES IS AN ENERGY-REDUCED DIET COMBINED WITH INCREASED PHYSICAL ACTIVITY.

> Losing weight and increasing levels of physical activity not only lower blood glucose levels and metabolic risk factors, but also improve general health and wellbeing.

This approach is endorsed by all health authorities globally. Scientific evidence consistently and repeatedly shows that for people who are overweight or obese, and who have pre-diabetes or type 2 diabetes, losing weight and increasing levels of physical activity not only lower blood glucose levels and metabolic risk factors, but also improve general health and feelings of wellbeing.

While dietary fads and novel exercise regimes abound in the popular media and may achieve temporary weight loss, our challenge at the CSIRO is determining – based on the **highest-quality scientific research** – the best diet and exercise approaches to optimise weight loss over the long term, and at the same time maximise the improvements in blood glucose control and reduce the metabolic risk factors for type 2 diabetes.

For some, adopting lifestyle changes can be a challenge, so our goal is to provide an easy step-by-step guide to help improve your lifestyle, combined with a diet and exercise plan that will provide you with larger effects and greater improvements for your efforts than traditional approaches.

A TRADITIONAL *dilemma*

In the past, based on the expert opinion at that time, the traditional one-size-fits-all dietary approach recommended by many health professionals and governing health bodies to achieve weight loss and normalise blood glucose levels in individuals with type 2 diabetes was an energy-reduced diet that was qualitatively no different to the Australian Dietary Guidelines for healthy eating.

This approach recommended a high intake of unrefined carbohydrate foods that are low-GI, fibre-rich and contain no added sugar, including wholegrain breads, cereals, starchy vegetables, pasta, legumes (beans and lentils) and fruits. It was recommended that up to 50 per cent of an individual's total energy intake came from these carbohydrates, spread evenly across the day.

Other health bodies around the world recommended carbohydrate intakes in the range of 45–65 per cent of the daily total energy, with some even higher than that! In practice, this meant that on a daily basis, an individual often consumed in excess of 45 grams of unrefined carbohydrate-based foods at each meal, and 15–30 grams as snacks, providing more than 220 grams of carbohydrate each day. (In terms of bread, which provides about 15 grams of carbohydrate per slice, this translates to 14 slices a day!)

Today, dietary guidelines for type 2 diabetes management still apply the generic principles of healthy eating recommended by the Australian Dietary Guidelines for all people (regardless of whether or not they have diabetes, high blood pressure or high blood cholesterol levels), and suggest eating at least 130 grams of low-GI, high-fibre and unrefined carbohydrates each day.

The suggested higher carbohydrate intake of the past was based largely on the recommended limits for total fat and protein intake. This stated that total fat should contribute less than 30 per cent of total energy intake, with the emphasis on including alternative substitutes for saturated fat – so that saturated fat provides under 10 per cent, and monounsaturated and polyunsaturated fat 10–20 per cent, of total daily energy. The recommendations suggested that for people who are overweight or obese, a fat intake below 30 per cent may promote better weight loss.

The low-fat recommendations also suggested that protein should contribute only 10–20 per cent of total energy intake. These recommendations have often seen modest results in weight and health changes that reduce the risk factors for type 2 diabetes, with many individuals still progressing to the need for diabetes medications to achieve improved blood glucose control.

For some time, the dilemma has been that type 2 diabetes management practices were not keeping up with the science, with emerging evidence demonstrating that carbohydrate restriction – with higher intakes of lean protein and healthy unsaturated fats – improves blood glucose control, reduces glucose levels and fluctuations across the day and improves blood fat profile, even without weight loss.

This is partly because dietary carbohydrates are made up of glucose molecules, meaning carbohydrate-rich foods all digest down into large amounts of glucose, making it harder to control blood glucose levels. Excess dietary glucose is also turned into triglycerides by the liver, which can be reduced by restricting dietary carbohydrate (and therefore glucose).

For some time, the dilemma has been that type 2 diabetes management practices were not keeping up with the science.

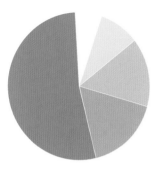

Current eating patterns
of Australians

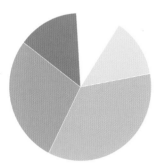

Traditional higher-
carbohydrate, moderate-
protein, low-fat diet

The CSIRO Low-carb Diet

- Carbohydrate
- Protein
- Monounsaturated fat
- Polyunsaturated fat
- Saturated fat

Towards a NEW UNDERSTANDING

While a traditional higher-carbohydrate (unrefined), moderate-protein, low-fat diet remains a commonly adopted approach for managing obesity and type 2 diabetes, extensive research suggests that this approach is only associated with modest weight loss, reductions in metabolic risk factors for type 2 diabetes and improvements in blood glucose control, particularly in people with type 2 diabetes.

In fact, research by the CSIRO and other internationally respected teams has advanced our understanding of the effects of dietary carbohydrate, protein and fat on metabolic risk factors and blood glucose control.

Collectively, this research suggests that the level of carbohydrate in traditional dietary approaches may be too high, particularly with the current high levels of physical inactivity and excessive weight in our society today. This is especially the case for people with insulin resistance or risk factors for type 2 diabetes, or those with type 2 diabetes, which represents a large portion of individuals.

Indeed, this research suggests that restricting the amount of carbohydrate in the diet, and increasing the proportion of energy from protein and unsaturated (healthy) fats – irrespective of whether an individual loses weight – will result in greater improvements in blood glucose control, by lowering blood glucose levels, reducing the rises in blood glucose levels after eating, and better stabilising the blood glucose profile through the day. In addition, this style of eating will also promote greater reductions in the metabolic risk factors for type 2 diabetes and heart disease.

Based on more than 20 years of research by the CSIRO and other leading scientific institutions into the most effective nutrition principles for type 2 diabetes management, weight control, metabolic health and wellbeing, we created a nutritionally complete, energy-controlled eating plan that was **lower in carbohydrate and proportionally higher in protein and unsaturated fat** (including monounsaturated and polyunsaturated fats) – a plan that is now well known as the **CSIRO Low-carb Diet**.

This dietary profile is distinctly different to the traditional higher-carbohydrate, moderate-protein, low-fat diet, and to what many Australians living with type 2 diabetes are currently eating – but it is what the latest scientific evidence is clearly telling us is effective to reduce risk factors and improve type 2 diabetes management.

AND IT WORKS.

The CSIRO Low-carb Diet was tested rigorously in a randomised controlled trial by comparing its effects directly to a traditional higher-carbohydrate (unrefined), moderate-protein, low-fat diet in individuals with type 2 diabetes. These results have been published in several prestigious scientific journals including *Diabetes Care*, *The American Journal of Clinical Nutrition* and *Diabetes, Obesity and Metabolism*.

The RESEARCH TRIAL

In this clinical trial, 115 adults who were overweight or obese and had type 2 diabetes were randomly divided into two groups.

Group 1 followed an energy-reduced diet that was low in unrefined carbohydrate (good-quality), high in protein and unsaturated fat, and low in saturated fat – in other words, the CSIRO Low-carb Diet. Of the total daily energy allowance, 14 per cent of kilojoules came from carbohydrate, 28 per cent from protein, and the remaining 58 per cent from fat (with less than 10 per cent from saturated fat).

Group 2 followed a diet that provided the same amount of energy, but was high in good-quality unrefined carbohydrate (53 per cent), relatively low in protein (17 per cent) and low in fat (30 per cent, with less than 10 per cent saturated fat). This high-carb, low-fat approach has traditionally been recommended by leading health authorities, and is similar to what many Australians are typically eating.

Both study groups also participated in the same structured physical activity program, undertaking the same 60 minutes of combined aerobic and resistance exercise three times a week.

WHICH HEALTH MARKERS WERE MEASURED?

Before and after the trial, each participant underwent a comprehensive health assessment to determine which diet approach worked better. This included recording their body weight and composition (to monitor changes in fat and lean body tissue), along with the metabolic risk factors that a GP would assess for diabetes and heart disease risk, including:

▶ blood pressure
▶ blood glucose control – including levels of fasting blood glucose and HbA1c, as well as the degree of blood glucose variability across the day
▶ the level of blood glucose–controlling medications each participant was using
▶ blood fat (lipid) profile, including triglyceride, LDL ('bad') cholesterol and HDL ('good') cholesterol levels.

Other health markers that can also be negatively affected by high blood glucose levels and diabetes were also assessed, including:

▶ kidney function
▶ mental health – including mental performance, mood and quality of life.

The health markers measured in the CSIRO trial

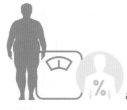
Obesity or body weight and composition

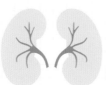
Blood pressure

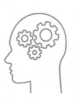
Blood glucose control including fasting blood glucose, HbA1c and blood glucose variability across the day

Blood glucose-controlling medications

Blood lipid profile

Kidney function

Mental health, mood and quality of life

HOW DID THE HEALTH OUTCOMES COMPARE?

After 1 year: It was found that both groups enjoyed substantial and similar reductions in body weight, fat mass, blood pressure, glycosylated haemoglobin (HbA1c) and fasting glucose (clinical measures of blood glucose control), and LDL cholesterol ('bad' cholesterol), as well as improved mood and quality of life. Both diets also had similar effects on cognitive (brain) function. The level of changes that occurred represent clinically relevant improvements in health and wellbeing that significantly reduce the risk of poor health outcomes. This may include reducing your risk of developing depression and other mental health disorders such as Alzheimer's disease.

Health measure	Average change in low-carbohydrate diet group	Average change in high-carbohydrate diet group
Body weight	-9.1% (10 kg)	-9.1% (10 kg)
Fat mass	-8.3 kg	-8.3 kg
Blood pressure	-6/-6 mmHg	-6/-6 mmHg
HbA1c	-1% (-12.6 mmol/mol)	-1% (-12.6 mmol/mol)
Fasting glucose	-1.4 mmol/L	-1.4 mmol/L
LDL cholesterol	-0.1 mmol/L	-0.2 mmol/L
Mood and quality of life	about 30% improvement	about 30% improvement

Interestingly though, there were striking differences between the two groups for several important health outcomes:

▶ The low-carb diet group experienced much greater reductions in their need for diabetes medication, a reduction that was twice as large as it was in the high-carb diet group.

▶ The low-carb group also had a greater reduction in blood glucose variation throughout the day, a reduction that was three times greater than in the high-carb group. These greater improvements meant that people in the low-carb group experienced a more stable blood-glucose profile throughout the day (in other words, the degree of excessively high and low blood-glucose levels was reduced). This means better blood-glucose control and lower risk of hypoglycaemia, reduced medication costs and fewer medication side effects. The reduced levels of blood-glucose variation means a lower risk of health complications associated with diabetes.

▶ The low-carb group also had much greater reductions in blood triglyceride levels and increases in HDL-cholesterol ('good' cholesterol) levels. This means greater improvement in heart health and lower risk of heart disease.

SIGNIFICANT ADDITIONAL BENEFITS OF LOW-CARB DIET

Health measure	Average change in low-carbohydrate diet group	Average change in high-carbohydrate diet group
Medication requirements*	−40%	−20%
Glycaemic variability	−30%	−10%
Blood triglycerides	−0.4 mmol/L	−0.01 mmol/L
HDL cholesterol	+0.1 mmol/L	+0.06 mmol/L

*Medications for controlling blood glucose levels

After 2 years: The benefits and differences in health outcomes between the two groups were maintained, and the number of people who completed the trial remained similar in both groups. The study also showed that both the low-carb and high-carb diet did not affect clinical markers of renal (kidney) function.

THE SIGNIFICANCE OF OUR RESULTS

Each change in one of the measures seen above has an important effect on our health.

▶ Average figures from large population studies show that people with a 5/5 mmHg lower blood pressure (say 135/90 mmHg compared to 140/95 mmHg) have a more than 30 per cent lower risk of stroke and 20 per cent reduction in the risk of dementia or heart failure, or dying from heart disease.

▶ In the same way, a drop in one unit of HbA1c (say from 7.5 per cent to 6.5 per cent, a 1 per cent decrease) reduces the risk of heart attack by 14 per cent, of developing microvascular disease by one-third, of limb amputation by almost half and of diabetes-related death by 21 per cent.

▶ And finally, for every 1 per cent increase in HDL cholesterol, the risk of heart disease falls by 3 per cent. The increase enjoyed by our trial participants following the low-carb diet and exercise plan was 8 per cent, which means a 24 per cent decrease in cardiovascular disease risk.

▶ The other major benefit of the diet and exercise plan was the large reduction in dependence on medications. In other words, by following the low-carb diet and exercise plan, you can be confident that you're becoming healthier, regardless of how much weight you lose.

Overall, these results confirm that **The CSIRO Low-carb Diabetes Diet & Lifestyle Solution** is not only an effective weight loss and management approach, but also offers superior benefits for improving blood glucose control and reducing heart disease risk factors, without concerns of negative impact on brain or kidney function.

So why and how DOES THE DIET WORK?

The CSIRO Low-carb Diabetes Diet & Lifestyle Solution works so well because it has been developed using the latest scientific evidence to create an eating pattern that provides an optimal amount and balance of macronutrients for weight and blood glucose control, metabolic health and wellbeing, to maximise the health benefits that can be gained – particularly for people with pre-diabetes or type 2 diabetes. In addition, it also takes into account the individual's need for diet flexibility.

1 **IT LIMITS CARBOHYDRATE AND HIGH-CARB FOODS**

Eating foods with higher amounts of carbohydrate – such as bread, cereals, rice, pasta, potatoes, many fruits, and foods high in sugar – can cause blood glucose levels to rapidly rise, which can increase the risk of type 2 diabetes and heart disease, along with the health consequences associated with these conditions. This is because all carbohydrates are broken down into simple sugars and released into the bloodstream as glucose.

As shown in the diagram below, high-carbohydrate foods such as bread and jam will give rise to higher blood glucose levels over a shorter time period (peak) with an equally fast drop, compared to foods that are relatively higher in dietary protein (lean meat, fish, chicken, tofu) and healthy fats (nuts, avocado and unsaturated oils).

EFFECTS OF FOODS RICH IN DIFFERENT MACRONUTRIENTS ON BLOOD GLUCOSE LEVELS OVER TIME

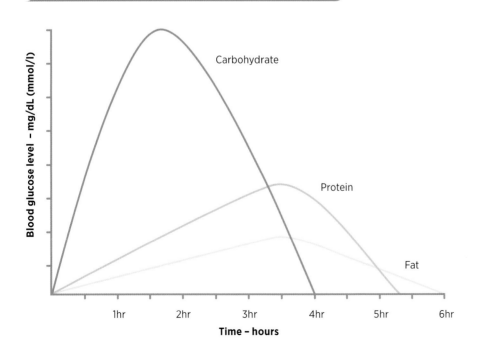

This is why a meal higher in carbohydrate and lower in fat and protein (such as a white-bread sandwich or toast, apple and a glass of juice) will produce greater blood glucose responses (a rapid spike and fall) compared to a meal with a lower amount of total carbohydrate, and higher levels of protein and fat (such as roast chicken with green vegetables, nuts and cheese), which results in a lower and more stable blood glucose level across the day.

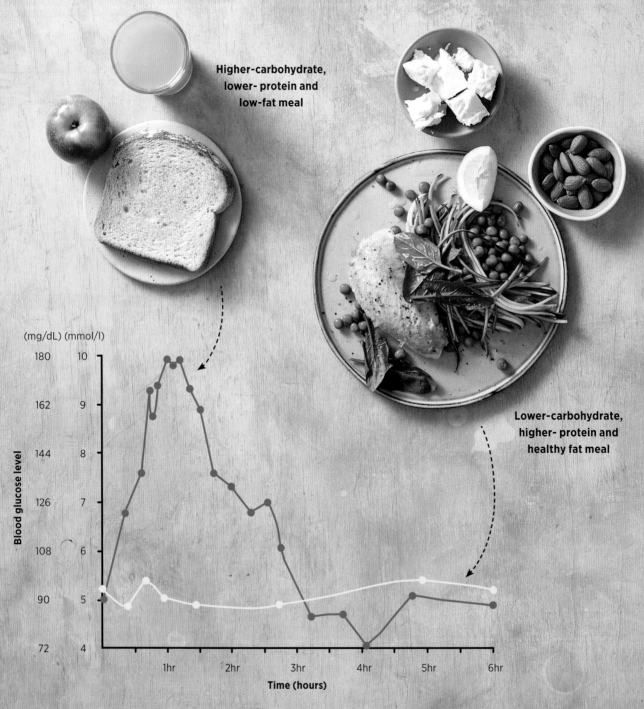

Higher-carbohydrate, lower- protein and low-fat meal

Lower-carbohydrate, higher- protein and healthy fat meal

Where do I find carbohydrates?

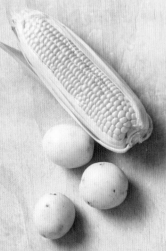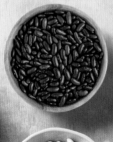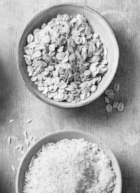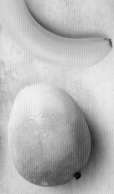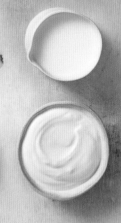

Starchy vegetables
Regular and sweet
potatoes, corn
(fresh or frozen)

Legumes
Lentils, beans
and peas

**Breads, cereals
and grains**
such as wheat, oats,
pasta and rice

Whole fruit
Fresh and frozen
whole fruits and canned
fruit in natural juice

Dairy
Milk and yoghurt

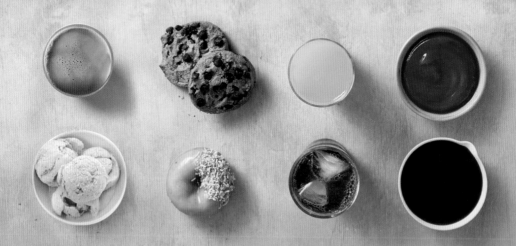

Other carbohydrate-containing foods
such as biscuits, cakes, sugary drinks and desserts
(including fruit juice, flavoured milk and ice creams),
sauces, jam and many other highly processed foods

Also, when it comes to carbohydrate, the higher the total amount of carbohydrate in a food or meal – and the more refined and highly processed that carbohydrate is – the more it will increase blood glucose.

The degree to which a food or meal will increase blood glucose levels is reflected in a measure known as glycaemic load (GL).

There are two factors that determine the level of glycaemic load: a food's **glycaemic index** (GI; in per cent), and the **total amount of carbohydrate** (G; in grams).

$$\text{GL} = \text{Type (GI\%)} \times \text{Quantity (G)}$$

The glycaemic index (GI) is a rating for food, based on the degree to which blood glucose will rise after eating. Foods are given a GI score of 1 to 100, based on the total rise in blood glucose after a reference amount is eaten, compared to pure glucose, which is set at 100.

▶ **Low GI** is up to 55.
▶ **Medium GI** is greater than 55 to 69.
▶ **High GI** is 70 and above.

In other words, the higher the GI scoring of a food, the higher and quicker it will raise blood glucose levels.

Based on the glycaemic load equation, it is clear that simply eating carbohydrate foods with a lower GI is a good strategy to help reduce the overall glycaemic load. However, the other part of the equation is the total amount of carbohydrate.

While both the GI rating and the total amount of carbohydrate play a role in determining the glycaemic load of a food and meal, it is clear that focusing on **reducing the total amount (quantity) of carbohydrate** (rather than the GI rating) will have the greatest impact on reducing the glycaemic load and blood glucose response after eating.

A good example to demonstrate this is presented below. A typical high-carbohydrate food is rice, with 1 cup of cooked rice providing about 60 grams of carbohydrate.

- A high-GI rice with a score of 72 per cent, multiplied by the 60 grams of carbohydrate in 1 cup of rice, equates to a GL score of **43**.
- This GL score can be lowered to a score of **26**, simply by choosing a rice option with a lower GI – in this case 43 per cent – and keeping the amount of rice in the meal the same.
- However, the GL score can be lowered strikingly (by ~74 per cent) to a score of **11**, simply by reducing the total amount of rice to ¼ cup (or 15 grams of carbohydrate), even if the high-GI rice (with a GI score of 72 per cent) is still used.
- This score can be lowered even further by selecting the low-GI rice option. Using ¼ cup of rice with a GI of 43 per cent will give a GL score of about **6.5**.

This clearly demonstrates that reducing the amount of high-carbohydrate foods and the total amount of carbohydrate in a meal and the diet will have the largest effect in reducing the glycaemic load and blood glucose response after eating, making it easier to also achieve more stable blood glucose levels throughout the day. This may also mean that you do not need as much medication to control your blood glucose if you have type 2 diabetes.

Research has also consistently shown that reducing the total amount of carbohydrate in the diet also **helps reduce blood triglyceride levels** – which is why a low-carbohydrate diet can be effective in people with the diabetes risk factor of high blood-triglyceride levels.

Other recently published research further supports the benefit of carbohydrate-restricted diets in people with type 2 diabetes, and the findings shown in our CSIRO trial. A recent meta-analysis – a combined analytical summary of several good-quality clinical trials – showed that compared to a traditional high-carbohydrate, low-fat diet, consuming a diet with low to moderate amounts of carbohydrate had greater effects on improving blood glucose control in people with type 2 diabetes – and indeed that the greater the level of carbohydrate restriction, the greater the improvement in blood glucose control.

Glycaemic load of rice

HIGH-GI, 1 CUP SERVE:
72% X 60 G = 43

LOW-GI, 1 CUP SERVE:
43% X 60 G = 26

HIGH-GI, ¼ CUP SERVE:
72% X 15 G = 11

LOW-GI, ¼ CUP SERVE:
43% X 15 G = 6.5

② IT INCREASES THE AMOUNT OF 'HEALTHY' UNSATURATED FAT

For quite some years we were told that a diet low in fat was the best for all of us. However, a wide body of high-quality research now suggests that a blanket low-fat message may not be the answer, and clearly shows that all fats are not equal – and that it is the fat *quality* rather than *quantity* that is most important. In fact, within an energy-controlled eating plan, having a higher amount of unsaturated fats, actually improves heart health and reduces metabolic risk factors. Unsaturated fats, including monounsaturated and polyunsaturated fats, are found in nuts, seeds, oils (olive, canola, sunflower, peanut and sesame), avocados, olives, and oily fish such as salmon and tuna – all of which are included in *The CSIRO Low-Carb Diabetes Diet & Lifestyle Solution*.

> A wide body of high-quality research now suggests that a blanket low-fat message may not be the answer.

Research shows that consuming these types of fats:

▶ improves insulin sensitivity (reduces insulin resistance), producing a lower blood glucose response

▶ reduces total blood cholesterol, LDL ('bad') cholesterol and triglyceride levels

▶ increases HDL ('good') cholesterol levels

▶ improves the functioning of the blood vessels in the heart.

Having a higher amount of unsaturated fat in meals also helps to further reduce the blood glucose rises of any carbohydrate in the meal. It does this by slowing the process of digestion and the release of carbohydrate from the stomach to the bloodstream.

③ IT KEEPS THE AMOUNT OF 'UNHEALTHY' SATURATED FATS LOW

Saturated fats are typically found in foods such as butter, lard (pig fat), tallow (beef fat) and coconut oil, and in high quantities in processed and 'discretionary' or 'junk' foods like pastries, biscuits, cakes and pies. In an opposing manner to unsaturated fat, saturated fats have been shown to increase LDL ('bad') cholesterol levels in the blood, increasing the risk of heart disease. A number of studies have also shown that replacing saturated fat with monounsaturated and polyunsaturated fat can reduce the risk of heart disease. There is growing debate about whether saturated fat in itself is bad for us, and some recent studies have even disputed any association with saturated fat intake and risk of heart disease or type 2 diabetes.

However, clinical evidence from randomised controlled studies has shown that high intakes of saturated fat could increase the risk of heart disease and type 2 diabetes by:

▶ promoting insulin resistance

▶ elevating LDL ('bad') cholesterol, which can harden the walls of the arteries

▶ impairing blood vessel function, particularly in the heart.

In view of this uncertainty, it may still be a good idea to limit your intake of saturated fat (with the exception of saturated fat from most dairy foods, which does not appear to increase risk of heart disease), or to replace foods high in saturated fat with small amounts of foods containing unsaturated fats. For this reason, *The CSIRO Low-carb Diabetes Diet & Lifestyle Solution* has been designed to limit the saturated fat content to no more than 10 per cent of total energy intake.

Overall, *The CSIRO Low-carb Diabetes Diet & Lifestyle Solution* takes advantage of the different effects of the fat types, by providing a higher proportion of energy from monounsaturated and polyunsaturated fats to deliver these benefits, while keeping saturated fat intake low. This enables optimal blood glucose control, while also improving heart health.

Fats in food

Saturated fat

Meat: chicken skin, processed meats, mince, fatty meat cuts including marbled red meats

Baked goods: cakes, biscuits, sweet and savoury pastries, pies

Takeaway foods: pizza, burgers

Fats: butter, cream, ghee, coconut oil, palm oil

Polyunsaturated fat

Omega-3

Fish: salmon, sardines

Nuts and seeds: flaxseeds

Omega-6

Nuts and seeds: walnuts, pine nuts, pecans, Brazil nuts, sunflower seeds

Oils: sunflower oil, sesame oil

Soy beans

Monounsaturated fat

Avocados

Nuts and seeds: almonds, cashews, macadamias, hazelnuts, pecans, peanuts

Oils: olive oil, canola oil

Meats: lean fish and chicken

Olives

4 IT INCREASES THE AMOUNT OF PROTEIN

A higher intake of dietary protein offers several important benefits for type 2 diabetes management and weight control. It can:

▶ improve body composition by maintaining a higher amount of lean muscle tissue, particularly when combined with exercise training; this will maintain a higher resting metabolic rate and total energy expenditure, making it easier to maintain a lower body weight
▶ help us burn more energy from processing and digesting food, also making it easier to maintain a healthy body weight
▶ help control our appetite and the amount of food we eat, as it increases the feeling of fullness of eating – again making it easier to maintain a healthier, lower body weight.

Protein in our meals also further helps to reduce the rise in our blood glucose levels from the carbohydrate in meals. Similar to fat, it does this by slowing the process of digestion and the release of carbohydrate from the stomach to the bloodstream.

5 IT IS NUTRITIONALLY COMPLETE

The CSIRO Low-carb Diabetes Diet & Lifestyle Solution differs from many other low-carb diets because it includes foods from all major food groups, with a focus on core, nutrient-dense whole foods, ensuring the diet contains all the essential vitamins, minerals, trace elements and fibre needed for good health.

Leading health authorities now support low-carbohydrate diets for type 2 diabetes management

The strong growing body of scientific research demonstrating the advantages of a low-carb diet in lowering blood glucose levels and improving metabolic health has created much international debate among leading health professionals, governing health authorities and the public about the most appropriate dietary approaches for managing pre-diabetes and type 2 diabetes.

This research continues to challenge the traditional recommendation of a high unrefined carbohydrate, low-protein, low-fat diet as the only dietary approach, and is leading a global paradigm shift in clinical practice guidelines for managing type 2 diabetes that has seen a growing acceptance of low-carb diets as an effective dietary plan and treatment option.

In fact, the guidelines and position statements of several leading health authorities – including the American Diabetes Association, Diabetes UK, Diabetes Australia, Dietitian Association Australia (DAA) and the British Dietetic Association – have been recently amended and updated to acknowledge and support the role of low-carbohydrate diets as part of an individualised approach in the management of type 2 diabetes.

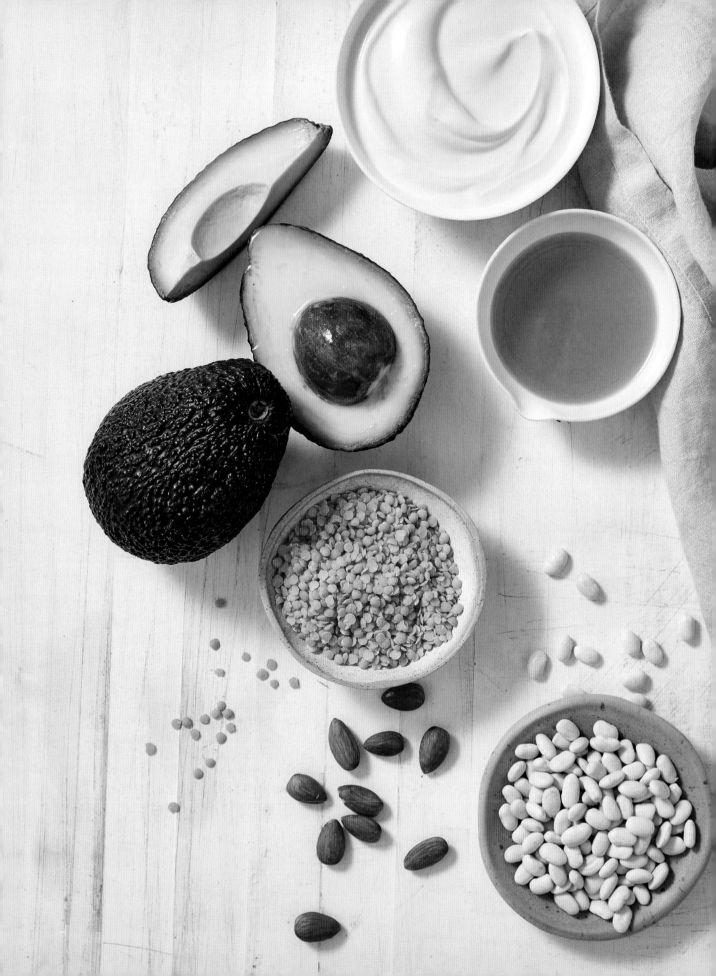

What about 'fasting' and very low-calorie diets?

As with low-carbohydrate diets, a large amount of high-quality research is starting to become available about 'fasting' dietary programs, informed by the latest scientific knowledge of effective nutrition strategies and solutions for weight and type 2 diabetes management. This research has resulted in considerable interest in, and popularity of, other dietary solutions such as intermittent fasting, alternate-day fasting and rapid weight loss that contravene traditionally recommended dietary practices.

Intermittent fasting, such as the 5:2 diet, involves restricting energy intake on 2–3 non-consecutive days per week, and eating 'freely' or 'normally' on the other non-restriction days. Alternate-day fasting is similar to intermittent fasting, but consists of a 'fast day' (only eating 0–25 per cent of your daily energy needs), alternating with a 'feed day' of eating freely without any restriction.

Current research in overweight or obese individuals, both with and without type 2 diabetes, suggests that both intermittent fasting and alternate-day fasting provide similar weight-loss results and improvements in health outcomes, including factors for heart health, diabetes risk and blood glucose control, compared to traditional dieting approaches of reducing your caloric intake every day. Although they provide potential alternatives, more studies in people with type 2 diabetes over longer periods of time are required to understand the full effects of these approaches.

Very low-calorie diets that provide no more than 800 kcal/day (~3500 kilojoules/day) are a strategy used for obtaining rapid weight loss.

In 2018, a study in people who were overweight or obese with type 2 diabetes showed that, compared to standard diabetes care from their GP, embarking on a rapid weight-loss diet was a more effective way of losing weight.

Results from this study also confirmed the benefits of weight loss for improving diabetes control – the more weight people lost, the more likely they were to be able to control their blood glucose levels without medication. In fact, 85 per cent of individuals who lost 15 kg or more were able to put their diabetes into remission: their HbA1c levels were below the type 2 diabetes classification cut-off, and they no longer required any diabetes medication.

Overall, emerging scientific findings suggest that intermittent fasting, alternate-day fasting or rapid weight-loss approaches could be used as alternative diet strategies to traditional daily moderate calorie restriction for weight loss, type 2 diabetes risk reduction and management of type 2 diabetes.

It is important to remember that one diet approach does not fit all – but just like *The CSIRO Low-carb Diabetes Diet & Lifestyle Solution*, these strategies offer effective alternative diet approaches to consider for weight and type 2 diabetes management.

However, as with any new changes to your current dietary and exercise habits, it is strongly recommended that if you want to try these approaches, you do this in close consultation with your healthcare team (particularly if you are taking medication) to ensure you achieve the best results in a safe and effective way.

Diabetes and kidney disease

Diabetes is a major risk factor for kidney disease. The high and fluctuating blood glucose levels can damage the vessels and nerves in the kidney, making it difficult for the kidneys to clean the blood properly, and making it difficult to empty the bladder. A high-protein diet is believed to place excessive strain on the kidneys, leading to poor kidney function; however, research suggests this is only the case for extremely high protein intakes – those that are much higher than is recommended in *The CSIRO Low-carb Diabetes Diet & Lifestyle Solution*. Although the proportion of energy from protein in the CSIRO Low-carb diet is higher than in a traditional high-carb, low-fat diet, the total amount of dietary protein is similar to that in the typical Australian diet – about 100 grams per day.

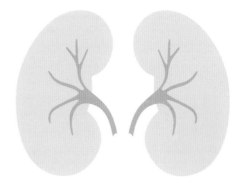

Our research showed that both *The CSIRO Low-carb Diabetes Diet & Lifestyle Solution* and a traditional high-carb, low-protein, low-fat diet had similar effects on kidney function in people who were overweight or obese with type 2 diabetes.

This result was also confirmed by a 2018 systematic review (a combined analysis of several research studies, considered a gold-standard approach to interpreting scientific literature) across 12 different studies of almost 1000 patients with type 2 diabetes – including some patients with early-stage kidney disease.

This analysis showed no differences in the effects on several measures of kidney function between a low-carb diet, and a control diet with a higher proportion of carbohydrate.

Based on these results, we can confidently say that *The CSIRO Low-carb Diabetes Diet & Lifestyle Solution* will maintain kidney function in people, including those with type 2 diabetes who do not have pre-existing kidney disease.

However, it is still important to start *The CSIRO Low-carb Diabetes Diet & Lifestyle Solution*, or any new nutrition plan, in close consultation with your healthcare team, so they can monitor your kidney health. This is particularly important if you already have type 2 diabetes and/or known kidney impairment, or poor kidney function, irrespective of whether you are starting a new diet plan or not.

Your HEALTHCARE TEAM

If you have type 2 diabetes, having a healthcare team to help you to understand, manage and control your symptoms, and also provide ongoing care throughout life, is important. Many people can be part of your healthcare team to help you live well with type 2 diabetes. The team will vary depending on your stage of diagnosis and the symptoms you experience, but you are the most important member of the team. Your role in your care is vital, as you will be making the day-to-day decisions about your diabetes – and the more you know about it, the easier it will become for you.

For example, a person newly diagnosed with diabetes will gain the greatest benefit from seeing the entire team to understand how diabetes expresses itself over time, and also how best to manage your medications, diet and exercise to prevent worsening of the disease. As you become more aware of what diabetes means to you, and how your lifestyle can be adapted to improve your self-care, you may work with a smaller team to help you prevent certain symptoms of the disease, or to specifically work on areas you may have challenges with, such as dietary management.

If you are newly diagnosed, in the short term, your medical management with your GP and/or endocrinologist (diabetes specialist) will be to focus on safely bringing your blood glucose levels under control, aiming to minimise daily blood glucose variations (highs and lows). They will also make sure your blood pressure and blood cholesterol levels are managed.

In the longer term, medical management treatments are aimed at preventing or slowing the progression of the disease to reduce your risk of complications. These complications are grouped together as macrovascular diseases of the large blood vessels, such as heart attack and stroke; and microvascular diseases of the small blood vessels, which involve poor circulation to organs and limbs, such as eye disease, kidney failure and nerve damage.

These strategies are centred around **long-term dietary management** with an accredited practising dietitian; **physical activity management** with an accredited exercise physiologist; and **medication management** with your GP. A credentialled diabetes educator (CDE) may also work with you to achieve **weight, cholesterol and blood pressure management** as needed. That is why incorporating a lifestyle modification plan such as *The CSIRO Low-carb Diabetes Diet & Lifestyle Solution* into this approach can be really effective, because **research clearly shows this plan is very effective at improving all of these health targets**.

Given that diabetes frequently goes undiagnosed in the community – with an estimated 500,000 with undiagnosed type 2 diabetes in Australia – we urge you to ask your GP to check your blood glucose levels each year. If you already have diabetes, your healthcare team will need to monitor your blood pressure, blood glucose and blood cholesterol levels regularly. Your healthcare team should always encourage you to learn how best to manage and control your diabetes yourself (under their supervision). If you find your healthcare team doesn't support you in this way, perhaps seek a second opinion, or a GP who can support you in making lifestyle changes.

> Your role in your care is vital, as you will be making the day-to-day decisions about your diabetes.

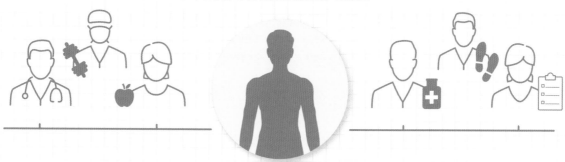

Patient-centred care:
THE PEOPLE IN YOUR TEAM

Reaching out for support can be a knowledge-gathering exercise, including learning who to contact and how best to access them. When it comes to self-care, speaking to those with skills and expertise in the area of diabetes is crucial for safe and effective diabetes management.

✚ YOUR GP (FAMILY DOCTOR)

Your GP is the first person you will see to discuss your symptoms and explore a diabetes diagnosis. If you don't have a family GP, or you don't have one with whom you feel you can openly explore your symptoms, a new GP is definitely worth considering. Your GP will have a central role in your care, and is responsible for making referrals to the other health professionals you will need on board for the best possible support. If you have type 2 diabetes or if you are at risk of getting type 2 diabetes, this is very important.

Your GP can refer you to all or any of the following healthcare providers:

✚ ENDOCRINOLOGIST

An endocrinologist is a medical specialist who can offer expert advice on the complications of diabetes or complex management needs.

✚ PHARMACIST

If you are already taking medications to manage your blood glucose levels, or you need to start taking them, a pharmacist is important to help you understand the medications and how you can manage them – especially if you are taking a few different ones. Your GP may ask a pharmacist to take you through a home or in-pharmacy medication review.

DIETITIAN

An accredited practising dietitian (APD) with expertise in diabetes management can work with you to develop a personalised eating plan, or to adapt *The CSIRO Low-Carb Diabetes Diet & Lifestyle Solution* to suit your needs, including cooking for a family or adjusting serving sizes. Your GP can refer you to a dietitian, or you can find one in your area online at daa.asn.au/find-an-apd.

EXERCISE PHYSIOLOGIST

An accredited exercise physiologist (AEP) can help you tailor *The CSIRO Low-Carb Diabetes Diet & Lifestyle Solution* exercise plan – or develop an alternative exercise program – to suit your lifestyle and needs, and to help with any injuries or ailments. Your GP can refer you to an exercise physiologist for an individual or group exercise program. To find out more, visit essa.org.au/find-aep.

CREDENTIALLED DIABETES EDUCATOR

The role of a credentialled diabetes educator (CDE) is to help you understand the broad area of diabetes management and complications, and how to adopt the recommendations provided by others in your team in a systematic way that suits you and your environment (at home, at work, and socially). Again, your GP can refer you to a credentialled diabetes educator. To find out more, visit adea.com.au.

PSYCHOLOGIST OR PSYCHIATRIST

We understand being diagnosed with diabetes can be overwhelming. A psychologist or psychiatrist can help you cope with a diabetes diagnosis and work through any stresses you may experience when managing your blood sugar levels, or as you start to create your life with diabetes. Seeking support is important to help you maintain good health and quality of life. Again, your GP can refer you to someone for support, or you can visit online to find someone in your area: psychology.org.au/Find-a-Psychologist.

PODIATRIST

The role of a podiatrist is to check your feet for circulation issues, as foot ulcers are a common complication of poor glucose management in people with diabetes. To find a podiatrist in your local area, or to find out more, visit podiatry.org.au.

Speak with your GP if you have any concerns or want to learn more about living with type 2 diabetes. You can also ask your GP to refer you to any members of your broader healthcare team for additional support.

Can a low-carb diet help treat type 1 diabetes and gestational diabetes?

Type 1 diabetes was previously known as insulin-dependent, juvenile or childhood-onset diabetes. It is a disorder characterised by deficient insulin production by the pancreas, and requires daily administration of insulin to control blood glucose levels. The exact cause of type 1 diabetes is not understood, and it is not preventable with current knowledge.

Gestational diabetes is a form of diabetes that occurs during pregnancy, characterised by hyperglycaemia and blood glucose values above normal. Women with gestational diabetes are at an increased risk of complications during pregnancy and childbirth. They and their children are also at increased risk of future type 2 diabetes.

Given that these conditions are underpinned by high blood glucose levels, and given the strong demonstrated clinical effectiveness of a low-carbohydrate diet in improving blood glucose control in people with type 2 diabetes (and reducing their need for blood-glucose controlling medication, including insulin), it is not surprising that there has been great interest in the potential role of a low-carb diet for managing type 1 and gestational diabetes.

Anecdotally, some people with type 1 diabetes have reported benefits from eating a diet with reduced carbohydrate. However, to date there is insufficient high-quality evidence to show the effectiveness of low-carb diets for people with type 1 and gestational diabetes. Until further evidence becomes available, it is recommended that people with these diabetes sub-types should first consult their physician before trying this approach.

At this time, low-carb diets are also not recommended for anyone under the age of 18 years, or those with specialised nutritional requirements.

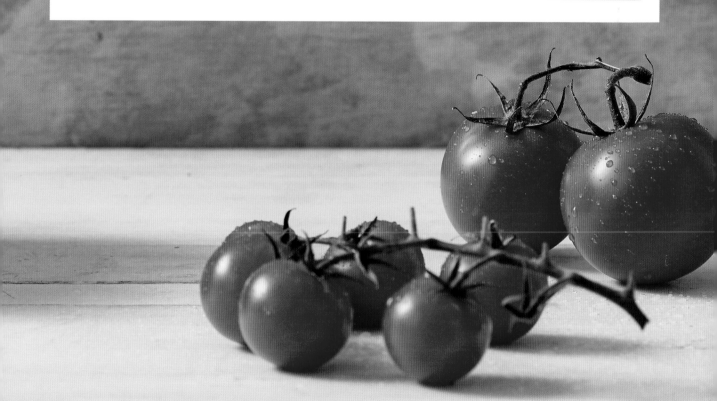

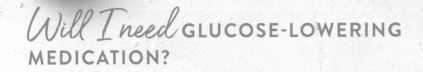

Will I need GLUCOSE-LOWERING MEDICATION?

For some, living with type 2 diabetes can mean being prescribed glucose-lowering medication, depending on the stage and severity of diabetes. Your GP or endocrinologist may prescribe glucose-lowering medications, or ask you to seek support from a wider network of health professionals (see pages 56–8) to help you reach your glucose control goals.

As you commence *The CSIRO Low-Carb Diabetes Diet & Lifestyle Solution*, there are good reasons why you will need to stay in close contact with your healthcare team, especially if you are taking oral hypoglycaemic agents or insulin.

If you are already taking medication for glucose control, it is very important that you seek a medication review prior to commencing a diet and exercise plan, and at least within the first two weeks of changing your lifestyle. Why? As you start to reduce your carbohydrate intake, or increase physical activity (with or without weight loss), the effect on your glucose levels can be profound, and you could see your blood glucose levels fall – and quite rapidly. This could result in you feeling a little dizzy, or even slightly hungry. Often this is misinterpreted as not eating enough, but in fact a modification and reduction to your medication regime by your GP can be all that you need.

Conversely, if you happen to do less exercise – perhaps due to illness, injury or holidays – then your blood glucose may rise again, and you will need to have your medication increased to manage during these times, even if you don't change your dietary intake.

Since low blood glucose levels can increase hunger and dizziness, especially if you are taking medications for diabetes control, you need to have a plan in place for dealing with these concerns. This is where your health professionals are essential.

For example, your GP can provide a hypoglycaemia (low blood glucose) management plan, explaining what levels your blood glucose need to be, and how to act when they aren't. In some cases, you may need to drink 100 ml of fruit juice to slightly increase your glucose level, or even use a HypoKit pen – a pen that injects glucagon, a hormone that opposes insulin and releases glucose from the liver to restore blood glucose levels. The pen is simple to use and can be easily administered by a friend, family member or even a bystander if you are unable to do this yourself.

MEDICATION MONITORING ON A LOW-CARB EATING PLAN

Research shows *The CSIRO Low-carb Diabetes Diet & Lifestyle Solution* is an effective option in lowering blood glucose levels, and can help many people reduce their need for medication, making it clinically inexpensive and lowering the cost to the individual and healthcare system.

When you are following a low-carbohydrate diet, your healthcare team needs to be confident in adjusting your diabetes medications accordingly, as your blood glucose levels are likely to fall substantially. To help them determine if any changes are needed to your medication management, what you will need to do is:

1. advise your team of the diet plan you are planning to follow, and how this is different to your previous diet and physical activity levels. This will tell them how much carbohydrate you are planning to consume. We recommend taking *The CSIRO Low-carb Diabetes Diet & Lifestyle Solution* with you to your appointment;

2. take your medications and scripts to the appointment with you, so you can discuss their changes and make notes on the packages as a reminder.

Remember that changes to your prescribed medication can only be managed by your GP and/or endocrinologist, and require a GP assessment.

During a period of medication review, it can be useful for you to self-monitor your blood glucose levels in a structured way – including immediately before each meal, and 2 hours afterwards, so you can communicate any changes in blood glucose levels to your healthcare team. This information will help them determine whether medications need to be adjusted further.

OVERVIEW OF KEY MEDICATIONS AND CONSIDERATIONS WHEN STARTING A LOW-CARB DIET

Diabetes medication (by drug group)	Risk of hypoglycaemia?	Considerations
Sulphonylureas (gliclazide) and **meglitinides** (repaglinide)	Yes	You will need to see your healthcare team, starting with your GP. You may be able to stop or gradually reduce the medication, with your team's monitoring
Insulin	Yes	You will need to see your GP to assess your ability to produce insulin. You may be able to stop or reduce your insulin with their guidance
SGLT2 inhibitors (farxiga, jardiance)	No	You will need to see your GP to assess your ability to produce insulin. You may be able to stop or reduce your medication with their guidance
Biguanides (metformin)	No	Your GP will assess the pros/cons of stopping or reducing
GLP-1 agonists (-enatide/-glutide)	No	Your GP will assess the pros/cons of stopping or reducing
Thiazolidinediones (glitazones)	No	Your GP will assess; commonly stopped if you are managing to lower your carbohydrate restriction longer term
DPP-4 inhibitors (gliptins)	No	Your GP will assess; commonly stopped if you are managing to lower your carbohydrate restriction longer term
Alpha-glucosidase inhibitors (acarbose)	No	Your GP will assess; commonly stopped if you are managing to lower your carbohydrate restriction longer term

Adapted from Murdoch C, Unwin D, Cavan D, Cucuzzella M, Patel M. 'Adapting diabetes medication for low carbohydrate management of type 2 diabetes: a practical guide.' *Br J Gen Pract.* 2019 Jul;69(684):360–361

The benefits of REAL-TIME CONTINUOUS BLOOD GLUCOSE MONITORING

One of the superior advantages of *The CSIRO Low-Carb Diabetes Diet & Lifestyle Solution* is its ability to improve your blood glucose profile and make it more stable, by minimising blood glucose fluctuations throughout the day. In the past, people would monitor their blood glucose levels by taking finger-prick blood glucose samples multiple times throughout the day, which can be inconvenient and invasive.

However, this is no longer the case with the availability of non-invasive, wearable continuous blood glucose monitoring devices. These devices have a small discreet glucose-measuring unit (about the size of a 50 cent coin) and a sensor filament that sits just beneath the skin and measures blood glucose levels every 5 minutes around the clock for up to 7–10 days. These devices allow the wearer to track their blood glucose profile 24 hours a day.

Some devices capture the information into the sensor, and this information can be downloaded and reviewed, showing when and how much your blood glucose levels went up and down throughout the day.

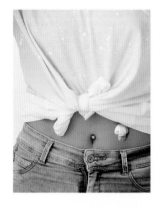

This will help you better understand how different foods, drinks and medication can affect your blood glucose profile, and what you were doing at a certain point in time to make your blood glucose have that response.

Alternatively, other devices can send the information in 'real time' to a smart phone, which means you can track your blood glucose profile 'live' and instantaneously. Having access to continuous glucose information provides feedback on the impact of your diet choices, exercise behaviours and medication on your blood glucose levels.

Using this type of technology when following *The CSIRO Low-carb Diabetes Diet & Lifestyle Solution* will enable you to directly see the benefits of this diet and exercise plan on stabilising your blood glucose profile throughout the day. This feedback can provide additional motivation and reinforcement of its many benefits, which can further help you stick to the plan and achieve greater health improvements. In fact, our research has demonstrated this very benefit.

In our 12-week clinical trial, 20 adults who were overweight or obese and had type 2 diabetes were randomly divided into two groups (see over the page).

> Having access to continuous blood glucose information provides feedback on the impact of your diet choices, exercise behaviours and medication on your blood glucose levels.

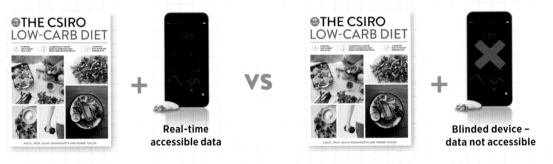

Real-time accessible data

Blinded device – data not accessible

Group 1 were provided with a copy of *The CSIRO Low-carb Diet* book and a real-time continuous blood glucose monitoring device, so they could see their blood glucose profile instantaneously and continuously while following the diet and exercise plan.

Group 2 were also given a copy of *The CSIRO Low-carb Diet* book and a real-time continous blood glucose monitoring device – except this time the device signal was switched off, so the user could not see their blood glucose profile.

Both study groups completed the program with limited additional professional instruction or support.

After just 12 weeks, participants in both groups lost about 7 kg and had a reduction in HbA1c levels of about 0.7 per cent (absolute units or 8 mmol/mol). These improvements were considered clinically relevant, meaning that they would translate to a significant reduction in the risk of diabetes-related complications – showing just how effective following the principles of *The CSIRO Low-carb Diet* by itself as a self-directed lifestyle program can be for improving your health.

In addition to these improvements, the group that had access to their real-time blood glucose information also experienced a **six times greater reduction in blood glucose variability**, and a **40 per cent greater reduction in diabetes medication requirements** compared to the group who wore the 'blinded' monitor and could not view their blood glucose profile. While this was only a small pilot trial, these results show that using a real-time continuous glucose monitor when following *The CSIRO Low-carb Diet* can reinforce the benefits of the program, and improve diabetes self-management behaviours that can lead to greater improvements in diabetes and blood glucose control.

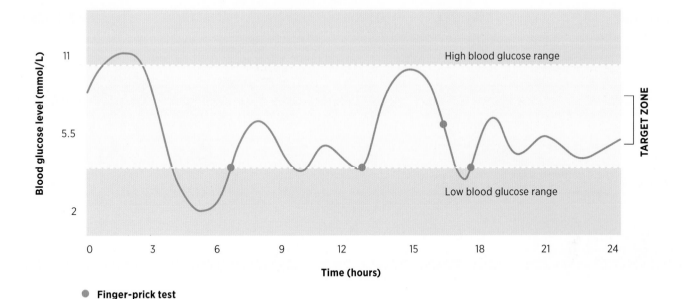

High blood glucose range

TARGET ZONE

Low blood glucose range

Blood glucose level (mmol/L)

11

5.5

2

Time (hours)

0   3   6   9   12   15   18   21   24

● **Finger-prick test**

As well as showing you the benefits of following *The CSIRO Low-carb Diabetes Diet & LIfestyle Solution*, a continuous glucose monitoring device can also detect large downward and upward swings in blood glucose levels, into the hypoglycaemia and hyperglycaemia ranges respectively. This information is extremely useful when adjusting medications, diet and exercise habits to prevent these swings.

The blue dots on the graph above record the results of finger-prick blood glucose tests, which would have provided no warning of these extremes, or even indicated that they had occurred.

Research suggests that self-monitoring your blood glucose levels using one of these dynamic devices is a really effective way of achieving better blood glucose control.

At the moment, these monitors are not cheap, but as they become more common, their prices will fall. The less expensive devices capture information into a recording unit that can be subsequently downloaded and viewed, costing typically between AU$50 and $100 per trace. The Bluetooth-enabled, real-time continuous glucose monitoring systems currently cost between $500 and $2000.

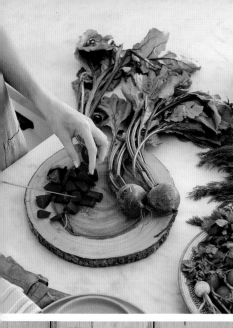
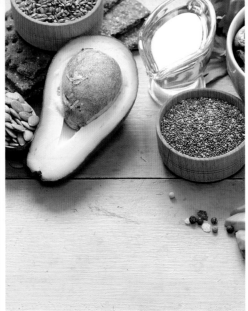
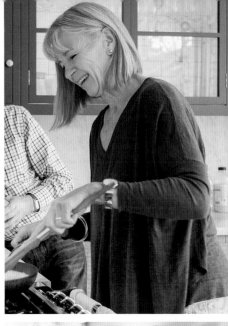
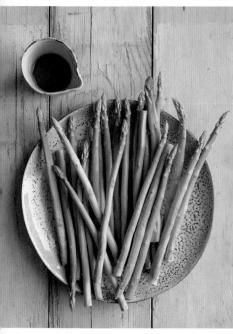

PART

3

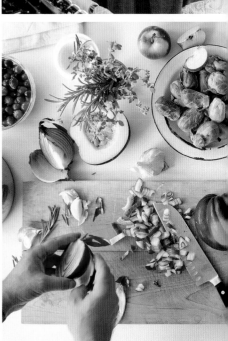
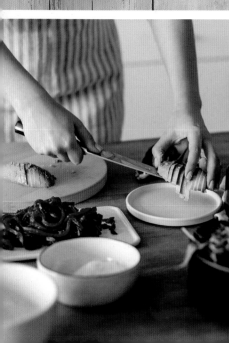
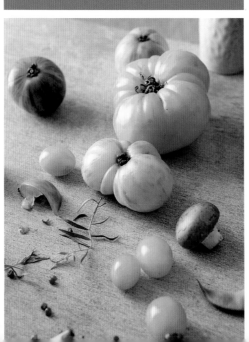
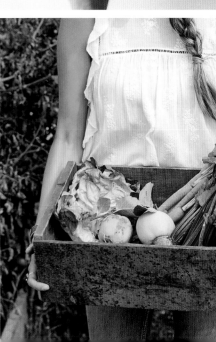

Following the
DIET & MEAL PLANS

The CSIRO Low-carb Diet and Meal Plans for Type 2 Diabetes

LET'S LOOK AT HOW TO USE THE CSIRO LOW-CARB DIET – IN CONJUNCTION WITH THE EXERCISE PLAN ON PAGES 266–79 – TO ACHIEVE THE GREAT BENEFITS IT CAN DELIVER.

The CSIRO Low-carb Diabetes Diet & Lifestyle Solution is an energy-controlled, nutritionally complete meal plan that focuses on eating nutrient-dense, whole core foods from all the key food groups, with the majority of the energy intake coming from healthy unsaturated fat and lean protein foods, with the inclusion of full-fat and low-fat dairy options.

Carbohydrate foods are included, with a focus on high-fibre, low-GI options that are high in resistant starch to promote bowel health. **This diet plan is not about saying no to carbohydrates**, but is instead about choosing **the right types** and **amount** across each day, to maximise the benefits for improving blood glucose and type 2 diabetes control. This plan includes **50 grams per day** of carbohydrate from high-fibre, low-GI foods.

How do I FOLLOW THE PLAN?

The most effective way to follow *The CSIRO Low-carb Diabetes Diet & Lifestyle Solution* is to first understand the foods and their food groups, and how these foods fit within your daily plan. Next, you will need to determine your individual energy requirements to ensure the plan you are following meets your own needs to help you achieve your personal goals.

The menu plans and recipes in this book are designed to help you understand how to spread your carbohydrate intake across the day, to help further control your blood glucose levels. Each recipe lists the number of food units from each food group per serve (see page 71 for food units required per day), as well as a 'carbohydrate flag' to show you how much carbohydrate it provides.

UNITS PER SERVE					
BREADS, CEREALS, LEGUMES, STARCHY VEGETABLES	DAIRY	LEAN MEAT, FISH, POULTRY, EGGS, TOFU	LOW-CARB VEGETABLES	MODERATE-CARB VEGETABLES	HEALTHY FATS
0	0	1.5	2	1	2

GRAMS CARB PER SERVE 10

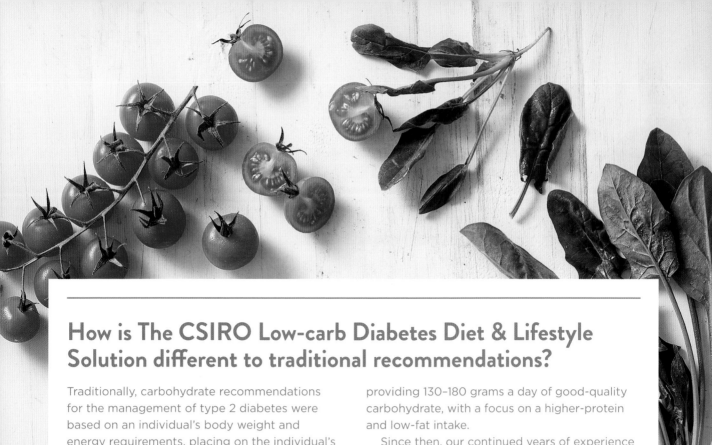

How is The CSIRO Low-carb Diabetes Diet & Lifestyle Solution different to traditional recommendations?

Traditionally, carbohydrate recommendations for the management of type 2 diabetes were based on an individual's body weight and energy requirements, placing on the individual's plate anywhere between 30 and 60 grams of carbohydrate at meals, and 15–30 grams for mid-meal snacks. This approach was designed to provide at least 200 grams of carbohydrate each day.

New scientific evidence has seen a shift in dietary guidelines towards lowering the carbohydrate intake to a minimum of 130 grams a day, which is classified as a moderate-carbohydrate diet.

Similar to these revised guidelines, when it was published 10 years ago, *The CSIRO and Baker IDI Diabetes Diet and Lifestyle Plan* book detailed a dietary plan based on providing 130–180 grams a day of good-quality carbohydrate, with a focus on a higher-protein and low-fat intake.

Since then, our continued years of experience and evolving research exploring the effects of dietary patterns and food responses in individuals with type 2 diabetes tells us that to better control blood glucose levels and manage feelings of hunger with a practical and realistic food approach, having an **even lower carbohydrate amount in the diet** is an important factor for success – along with **spreading meals across the day,** including core snacks, and considering carbohydrate extras as optional.

This has led us to develop *The CSIRO Low-carb Diabetes Diet & Lifestyle Solution*, and the eating plan detailed here.

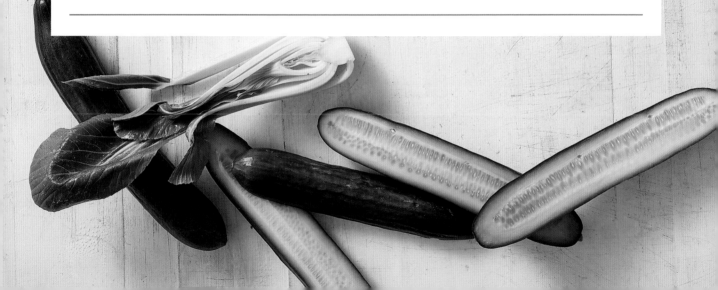

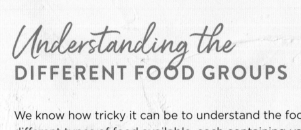

Understanding the
DIFFERENT FOOD GROUPS

We know how tricky it can be to understand the food groups, with so many different types of food available, each containing varying amounts of nutrients and energy. To make things easier, we have sorted foods into groups based on the **nutrients they provide** and assigned them a number based on **their energy content**. This will ensure you eat the right balance of nutrients for your energy requirements, while also providing you with a wide range of food options and possibilities.

The food groups table opposite shows the number of units of each food group you should eat each day, based on the energy level that is right for you. Generally, levels 1 and 2 are suitable for smaller or lower-weight individuals, while levels 3 and 4 are suitable for taller or higher-weight people. Instructions on how to determine your daily energy requirements are provided on page 74, so that you can select the correct energy level for you.

By eating the correct number of food units for your chosen energy level, spread evenly across each day, you are following **The CSIRO Low-carb Diabetes Diet & Lifestyle Solution**.

It is that simple.

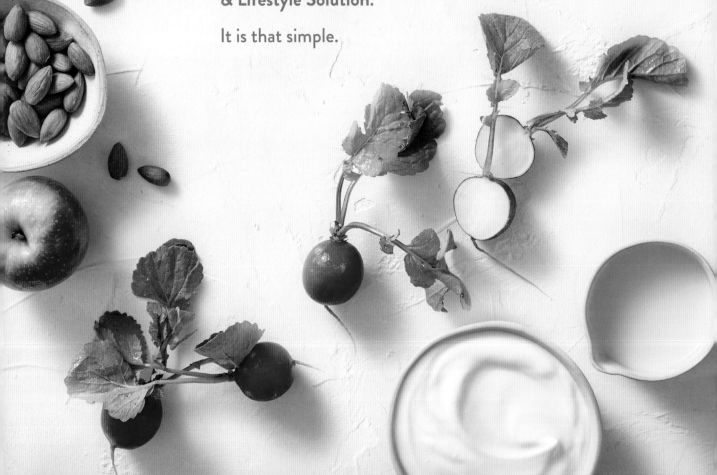

There are four energy levels to choose from, offering 6000–9000 kJ per day, that cater for most individual needs. Generally, levels 1 and 2 are suitable for women, while levels 3 and 4 are suitable for men. Please note that sometimes when building your own meals or menus using the units as a guide, you may have 'left-over' units, so we recommend using these remaining units as 'top-ups'.

Food groups for the diet	Level 1 (6000 kJ/day)	Level 2 (7000 kJ/day)	Level 3 (8000 kJ/day)	Level 4 (9000 kJ/day)	Key nutrients provided
Breads, cereals, legumes, starchy vegetables	1.5 units	1.5 units	1.5 units	1.5 units	Slow-release, low-GI carbohydrates, folate, fibre and B-group vitamins
Dairy	3 units	3 units	3.5 units	4 units	Protein, calcium, vitamin B12 and zinc. Dairy (except most cheeses) also contains carbohydrates.
Lean meat, fish, poultry, eggs, tofu	1 unit lunch 1.5 units dinner	1 unit lunch 2 units dinner	1 unit lunch 2.5 units dinner	1.5 units lunch 2.5 units dinner	Protein, zinc and vitamin B12. Red meats are highest in iron, fish in omega-3 fatty acids and pork in thiamin
Low–moderate carb vegetables	At least 5 units	At least 5 units	At least 5 units	At least 5 units	Minimal carbohydrates, and plenty of fibre, folate, vitamins A, B6 and C, magnesium, beta-carotene and antioxidants
Healthy fats	10 units	11 units	14 units	15 units	Vitamins A, E and K, antioxidants and omega-3 and omega-6 fats
Indulgences (optional)	2 units per week	2 units per week	2 units per week	2 units per week	Limited beneficial nutrients. Most contain added sugars, alcohol and/or saturated fats
Carbohydrate extras (optional) (Weeks 7+)	2 extras per day	2 extras per day	2 extras per day	2 extras per day	Carbohydrates. They also contribute vitamins and minerals as they come from your core food units

To choose which level is right for you ...

1.
Determine your daily kilojoule requirements for either weight loss or weight maintenance (see pages 74–5).

2.
Choose the level from the table above that fits these requirements.

3.
Look at the number of food units allowed within your level.

4.
Consult the daily food guide to see how this translates into a daily eating plan (see pages 79–83).

CARBOHYDRATE EXTRAS FOR LONGER-TERM MAINTENANCE AND FLEXIBILITY

Our experience tells us that the most effective way to follow *The CSIRO Low-carb Diabetes Diet & Lifestyle Solution* is to start with the baseline approach, which provides 50 grams of carbohydrate per day. After a few weeks you can, if you wish, increase your carbohydrate intake by 20 grams each day to a maximum of 70 grams per day – especially if you need slightly more carbohydrate over the longer term, or are simply trying to maintain your weight. We have included these carbohydrate 'extras' to create flexibility within our type 2 diabetes plan, so you can adjust your carbohydrate intake yourself or in consultation with your health professional to meet your personal needs.

Using the foods in the portions listed opposite, you can increase the intake of these foods by including up to 20 grams of carbohydrate (2 serves of extras) per day. It is still best to use the extra carbohydrate allowance as 'snacks' between meals, especially before you exercise. However, if you wish to add these to a meal, add them to meals that are already lower in total carbohydrate (see the 'carbohydrate flag' on each recipe), such as lunch or dinner.

During our research studies, some people indicated they were more satisfied and better able to maintain the dietary pattern in the longer term when they could increase their intake of low-GI, high-fibre carbohydrates to 70 grams each day. However, others preferred to stick to 50 grams because they found that increasing the carbs lead to progressive 'carb creep' and weight gain. Both are effective approaches, so select the strategy that is going to work best for you and give you the **best chance of sticking to the plan** while monitoring your progress by regular waist measurements, weighing and blood glucose checks.

As you introduce these 'carbohydrate extras', it is important to remember to measure your blood glucose about 2 hours after eating, so you can assess the effects the carbohydrate extras may be having on your blood glucose control. Even if you do not have type 2 diabetes, measuring your blood glucose will help you identify how your body is coping with the extra carbohydrates, and help you determine if you need them or not.

If you do not have type 2 diabetes, your body will be able to adjust more readily to the glucose being released from the carbohydrate extras, and you may not see the higher blood glucose levels a person with type 2 diabetes will see. Therefore, if your blood glucose, when measured, stays within the normal range (see page 19), you are fine to continue with the extras. However, be mindful that they also add an extra 500 kilojoules to your daily intake.

For those living with type 2 diabetes, by referring back to your diabetes management plan provided by your GP, you can check your blood glucose readings against those that have been recommended specifically for you, to determine if you are consuming enough or too little carbohydrate. It is important that you seek support from your healthcare professional if you are on medication, or you are not confident in assessing your level of blood glucose control.

Remember, the additional 20 grams of carbohydrate per day is entirely optional!

As you introduce these 'carbohydrate extras', it is important to remember to measure your blood glucose about 2 hours after eating.

CARBOHYDRATE EXTRAS 1 serving = 1 carb extra (10 g carb or less)

FRESH FRUIT –
choose most (can be included daily)

Apples	50 g
Apricots	2 medium
Bananas	40 g
Blueberries, frozen or fresh	60 g
Cherries	60 g
Feijoas	3
Figs	2
Kiwifruit	2 small
Lemon or lime juice, freshly squeezed (can add to sparkling water)	300 ml
Nectarine	1 small
Oranges	100 g
Passionfruit	7 (100 g)
Passionfruit pulp (no syrup)	50 g
Peach	1 small
Pears	50 g
Persimmon	1 small
Raspberries, frozen or fresh	100 g
Rhubarb (stewed, no added sugar)	400 g
Strawberries	200 g

DRIED FRUIT –
choose least (once or twice a week)

Apricots	20 g
Dates	2
Figs	1 (20 g)
Mixed dried fruit	10 g
Sultanas	10 g

OTHER

Vita-Weats, regular	2 biscuits (12 g)
Corn cakes/thins, multigrain	2 cakes (11 g)
Rice crackers (e.g. Sakata, Fantastic)	5 crackers (8 g)
Lentils, cooked and drained	80 g
Lentils, dried	15 g
Chickpeas, cooked and drained	40 g
Red kidney beans, cooked and drained	40 g
Four-bean mix, cooked and drained	40 g
Cannellini beans, cooked and drained	50 g
Mountain bread (wheat, rye and barley varieties)	½ regular rectangle
Fruit loaf	½ regular slice
Scone, wholemeal (commercial)	½ small scone (20 g)
Tortilla, corn	½ small
Wholegrain bread	½ regular slice
Low-fat yoghurt (Greek-style)	75 g
Reduced-fat evaporated milk (e.g. Carnation)	100 ml
Skim milk	100 ml
Green peas, cooked	120 g (¾ cup)
Sweet potato, cooked	50 g
Corn kernels, cooked	40 g or 2 tablespoons kernels

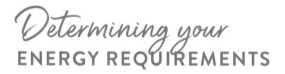

Determining your
ENERGY REQUIREMENTS

The first step is to calculate your estimated daily energy requirements. This will not only help to ensure the energy level of your diet plan is tailored to your personal needs so you can attain and maintain a healthy body weight, but will also tell you how much of each food group you should eat to achieve the right energy and nutrient balance for your body size and exercise levels.

DETERMINING YOUR DAILY KILOJOULE REQUIREMENTS

The following calculation was used in our scientific trial to personalise the diet to each participant's energy needs. It estimates your daily kilojoule requirements to maintain normal body function and keep your weight stable. This is known as your basal metabolic rate (BMR). To determine your BMR, use the appropriate formula from the table below.

FORMULAS FOR CALCULATING YOUR BASAL METABOLIC RATE

Age (years)	BMR equation	
	Women	Men
18–29	(62 x weight in kilograms) + 2036	(63 x weight in kilograms) + 2896
30–59	(34 x weight in kilograms) + 3538	(48 x weight in kilograms) + 3653
60 and over	(38 x weight in kilograms) + 2755	(49 x weight in kilograms) + 2459

Note: There are a few different methods for calculating BMR. We've used the Schofield equation.

Once you've determined your **BMR**, you need to multiply it by an **activity factor** from the table opposite.

This will allow you to estimate your total daily kilojoule requirements.

Activity level	Description	Activity factor	
		Women	Men
Sedentary	Very physically inactive (work and leisure)	1.3	1.3
Lightly active	Daily activity of walking or intense exercise once or twice a week and a sedentary job	1.5	1.6
Moderately active	Intense exercise lasting 20–45 minutes at least three times a week or an active job with a lot of daily walking	1.6	1.7
Very active	Intense exercise lasting at least one hour each day or a heavy, physical job	1.9	2.1
Extremely active	Daily intense activity (i.e. nonstop training, e.g. an athlete in training) or a highly demanding physical job (e.g. armed forces)	2.2	2.4

If you're a healthy weight, there's no need to reduce your energy intake, so the number you're left with now is your daily requirement, and you can use this to choose the level from the table on page 71.

If you need to lose weight, calculate your estimated daily kilojoule requirement as follows.

To reduce your weight by about 0.5 kilogram each week, you'll need to reduce your energy intake by 2000 kJ per day. Once you've calculated your total daily kilojoule requirements above, subtract 2000 from this number to determine how many kilojoules to eat each day to achieve weight loss, and therefore which of the four levels to choose.

To reduce your weight by about 1 kilogram each week, you'll need to reduce your energy intake by 4000 kJ per day. Calculate your total daily kilojoule needs as above and subtract 4000. This will tell you how many kilojoules to eat each day to achieve this weight loss and therefore which of the four levels to choose.

Note: If your chosen level isn't working, you can move between levels until you start to see the changes you desire. Many people hit a weight-loss plateau after an initial drop in weight. If this happens, you can switch to a lower level until you reach your target. Your dietitian and exercise physiologist can also help you to overcome a plateau.

How it works IN PRACTICE

Lynette is 56 years old and weighs 82 kilograms. She works part time as an office assistant and looks after her grandchildren two days a week. Lynette goes for a walk most days. This makes her activity factor 1.5. She chooses the appropriate formula from the table on page 74 and calculates her BMR like this:

✳ **BMR = (34 x weight in kilograms) + 3538**
        = (34 x 82) + 3538
        = 6326 kJ per day

To calculate her total daily kilojoule requirements, Lynette will multiply her BMR by her activity factor:

✳ **Total daily energy requirement = 6326 x 1.5**
                                            = 9489 kJ per day

This is the amount of energy Lynette needs to maintain her current weight.

Lynette is overweight and would like to start by losing about 0.5 kilogram a week. She'll therefore reduce her estimated total daily kilojoule intake by 2000 kJ per day:

✳ **Total dieting energy requirement = 9489 – 2000**
                                             = 7490 kJ per day

Lynette rounds this down to the nearest thousand, 7000 kJ per day, and will therefore start on level 2. If she's feeling too hungry or losing weight too rapidly, Lynette can move to level 3 (8000 kJ). If she's not losing weight, she can drop down to level 1 (6000 kJ).

Our clinical experience has shown that if your calculated energy requirements are greater than 9000 kJ a day, even by 2000–3000 kJ, following the level 4 diet will still result in significant health benefits.

MAINTENANCE IN THE LONGER TERM

Lynette reaches her weight-loss goal after six weeks, and her health has improved significantly. She decides she's enjoying the diet but would like to eat some fruit each day. As she's now on maintenance, she can have up to 70 grams of carbohydrates each day, instead of the standard 50 grams. To add another carbohydrate serve, she uses the carbohydrate extras table on page 73 to select a fruit portion.

Your daily food guide: HOW MUCH OF EACH FOOD YOU SHOULD EAT AND WHEN

Now that you have calculated your energy requirements, and identified the best energy level for your needs from the table on page 71 – including the number of food units you will need from each food group each day – the next step is to understand how much food in each group equates to 1 unit.

This is useful as it helps you to determine which foods – and what amount of each food – you can swap for each other within each group. Building your confidence and knowledge of these foods and how they work within the plan is essential in helping you to become consistent in your eating patterns and maintain the plan in the longer term. In our research trial, participants told us that in the beginning, having a narrow selection of foods to choose from helped them to regain control of their eating habits.

Let's walk through the plan. Let's say you are starting on level 1, with the 6000 kJ/day dietary template. Looking at the chart on page 71, you'll see that you need to consume 1.5 units from the 'Breads, cereals, legumes, starchy vegetables' group each day. Using the information listed on the daily food guide on page 79, this means you could, for example, select 30 grams of a suitable cereal (1 unit) and 50 grams of sweet potato (0.5 unit) on a given day. Alternatively, you could obtain your 1.5 units by combining the foods in that category however you like. For example, a combination such as 4 rye Cruskits (1 unit) and 80 grams of cooked, drained lentils (0.5 unit) could be consumed from this food group each day.

This is the great advantage of **The CSIRO Low-carb Diabetes Diet & Lifestyle Solution**: it offers a wide range of choice and flexibility, enabling you to create daily menu plans that suit your food and taste preferences.

By simply making sure that you eat the correct number of food units each day for the energy level selected, and using foods of the type and amount specified in the daily food guide, you can easily 'mix and match' your ingredients and daily menus, knowing you'll still be gaining the full benefit of *The CSIRO Low-carb Diabetes Diet & Lifestyle Solution*.

While 2 units of **indulgence foods** a week have been included in the plan, it is important to remember that these are completely optional. Try to start the plan by avoiding these foods for the first few weeks, or until you feel that they are no longer at the forefront of your mind. We also suggest scheduling these indulgence foods into your week; this way they won't become an everyday habit, but you will have the opportunity to enjoy them on special occasions or as a treat, so you won't feel like you are missing out.

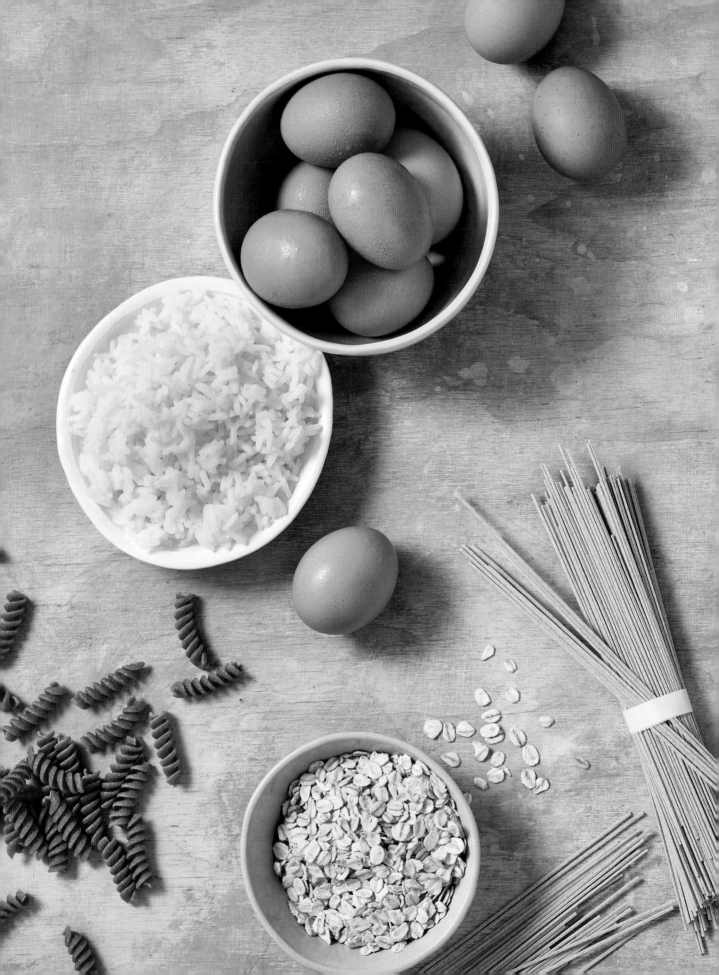

YOUR DAILY FOOD GUIDE FOR LEVEL 1 (6000 KJ)

The following pages give examples of the types and quantities of foods that can make up your daily intake of units on the diet.

Breads, cereals, legumes, starchy vegetables

1.5 UNITS A DAY
Opt for low-GI, wholegrain varieties high in resistant starch

1 UNIT HIGH-SOLUBLE-FIBRE, LOW-GI CEREALS
30 g suitable breakfast cereals, such as All-Bran, All-Bran Fibre Toppers, All-Bran Wheat Flakes, Freedom Barley + Muesli Cranberry, Almond and Cinnamon, Freedom Barley + Apple and Sultana, Hi-Bran Weet-Bix, untoasted natural muesli, raw natural rolled oats

1 UNIT BREADS
35 g multigrain bread
1 slice (45–50 g) Herman Brot Lower Carb bread
1 thin slice fruit bread
½ wholemeal pita bread (e.g. Mountain Bread wrap)
½ small wholemeal scone (25 g)
3 Ryvitas or 4 rye Cruskits
4 x 9-Grains Vita-Weats

1 UNIT LEGUMES
160 g cooked, drained lentils
80 g cooked, drained chickpeas or red kidney beans
100 g cooked, drained cannellini beans or four-bean mix

1 UNIT LOW-GI, HIGH-STARCH VEGETABLES
100 g sweet potato or potato (low-GI)
70 g corn

1 UNIT GRAINS
15 g wholemeal plain or self-raising flour, cornflour, rice flour, arrowroot or green banana flour
½ cup cooked soba noodles
½ cup cooked low-GI or wholemeal pasta
½ cup cooked quinoa or couscous
⅓ cup cooked low-GI rice

Dairy

3 UNITS A DAY
Where you see the choice of low-fat or reduced-fat, total energy and dietary calcium is being considered. Using full-fat versions are suitable, but just remember this may increase your total energy intake by 100–400 kJ. Also make sure you are choosing good sources of calcium (150 mg calcium per 100 g)

1 UNIT DAIRY IS EQUAL TO:
200 ml *plain* skim milk or low-fat cow's milk or calcium-enriched soy or almond milk
180 ml regular fat milk
20 g skim milk powder
100 g *plain* reduced-fat yoghurt or low-fat, lactose-free soy yoghurt
20 g cheddar, haloumi, parmesan, Swiss or feta cheese
55 g ricotta or cottage cheese
25 g mozzarella, bocconcini cheese or reduced-fat cream cheese

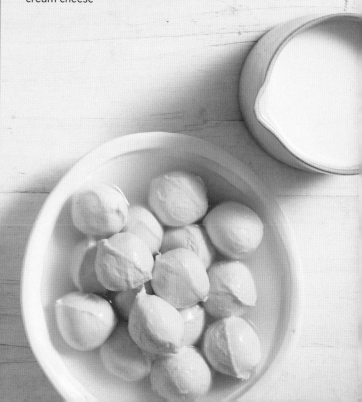

YOUR DAILY FOOD GUIDE FOR LEVEL 1 (6000 KJ)

Lean meat, fish, poultry, eggs, tofu

**2.5 UNITS A DAY (1 UNIT FOR LUNCH
+ 1.5 UNITS FOR DINNER)
Note: you can use 0.5 unit for breakfast;
if so, reduce to 0.5 unit for lunch**

**FOR LUNCH, CHOOSE FROM:
1 UNIT LEAN MEAT, FISH, POULTRY, EGGS, TOFU**
100 g (cooked weight) lean meat or fish: chicken, turkey,
    pork, beef, lamb or tinned or fresh fish or seafood
2 eggs (55 g/½ unit each)
100 g tofu (hard or silken)
We recommend fish for lunch at least twice a week
If you wish to have an egg for breakfast, just have 50 g
less meat at lunchtime to account for this

**FOR DINNER, CHOOSE FROM:
1.5 UNITS LEAN MEAT, FISH, POULTRY, EGGS, TOFU**
150 g (raw weight) lean meat or fish: chicken, turkey, pork,
    beef, lamb, fish or seafood
3 eggs (55 g/½ unit each)
150 g tofu
*We recommend fish for dinner at least twice a week and
red meat no more than three times a week*

Legumes are an excellent source of protein
for vegetarians or vegans, although they are
higher in carbohydrates than their animal-
based counterparts, so keep this in mind
when planning your daily intake
1 UNIT LEGUMES IS AS FOLLOWS:
160 g cooked, drained lentils (provides 15 g carbs
    and 11 g protein)
80 g cooked, drained chickpeas or red kidney beans
    (provides 12 g carbs and 6 g protein)
100 g cooked, drained cannellini beans or four-bean
    mix (provides 13 g carbs and 6 g protein)

Low–moderate carbohydrate vegetables

AT LEAST 5 UNITS PER DAY

CHOOSE FROM:

**1 UNIT LOW-CARBOHYDRATE VEGETABLES
(AT LEAST 3 UNITS OF THESE PER DAY)**

**150 G (1 CUP) UNCOOKED OR FROZEN (RAW) OF ANY
OF THE FOLLOWING VEGETABLES:**
artichoke (high in resistant starch), asparagus, bean
sprouts, bok choy, broccoli, broccolini, cabbage
(mustard and Chinese), citrus (lemon, lime, cumquat),
chillies, choy sum, cucumber, fresh herbs and spices,
garlic, kale, lettuce (all varieties), mushrooms, rocket,
spinach (English and baby), tomato, zucchini

**1 UNIT MODERATE-CARBOHYDRATE VEGETABLES
(MINIMUM 1 UNIT AND MAXIMUM 2 UNITS A DAY)**

**150 G UNCOOKED OR FROZEN (RAW) OF ANY OF THE
FOLLOWING VEGETABLES:**
bamboo shoots, broad beans, brussels sprouts,
cabbage, carrot, cauliflower, capsicum (all colours),
celery, eggplant, fennel, green beans, leek, onion,
parsnip, radish, snow peas, spring onion, swede turnip

**80 G (RAW OR FROZEN) MIXED BERRIES CAN ALSO
BE USED AS 1 MODERATE-CARB VEGETABLE UNIT;
CHOOSE ONLY FROM THE FOLLOWING:**
blackberry, blueberry, mulberry, raspberry, strawberry

**75 G (½ CUP) UNCOOKED OR FROZEN (RAW) OF ANY
OF THE FOLLOWING VEGETABLES:**
beetroot, green peas, pumpkin

Be careful to observe the smaller serving size

Healthy fats

1 UNIT HEALTHY FATS
1 teaspoon (5 g) oil, such as olive, grapeseed, flaxseed
  or sunflower oil
1 teaspoon (5 g) tahini (sesame butter) or cashew
  and other nut butters or pesto or curry paste
20 g avocado
1 tablespoon (20 g) hummus
1 teaspoon (5 g) Nuttelex margarine or canola margarine
10 g *unsalted* nuts (almonds, pecans, macadamias,
  walnuts, Brazil nuts, pistachios, pine nuts, sesame seeds,
  pumpkin seeds)
5 olives (20 g)
10 g almond meal
1 teaspoon (10 g) whole-egg mayonnaise

Indulgence foods (optional)

1 UNIT INDULGENCE FOOD, CHOOSE FROM:
Any food or drink providing approximately 450 kJ
  150 ml wine
  20 g chocolate
  40 g store-bought low-fat dips
  10 Arnotts Shapes
  1 x 20 g packet of chips
  10 Pringles
  ½ slice of pizza
  35 g hot chips

Pantry items that are FREE to use, daily!

Chilli, curry powder, balsamic vinegar, diet jelly,
diet topping, garlic, ginger, fresh lemon, fresh lime,
mustard powders or mustard creams, **oil-free**
dressings, fresh or dried herbs and spices, salt-
reduced stock, tomato salsas, Vegemite, vinegar,
unflavoured mineral or sparkling water, herbal teas
(no added sugar)

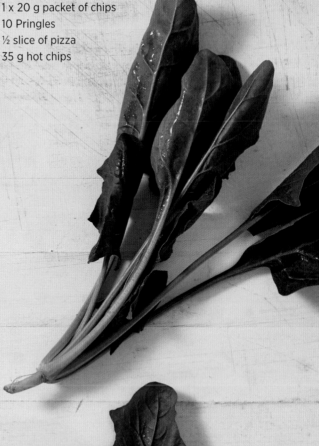

A SAMPLE DAY ON THE 6000 KJ DIET

Now that you understand the food groups, units and the portions and types of foods, the next step is to use them in your daily meals. You can follow the meal plans and recipes in this book, using the unit system to reach your daily unit totals for each food group. You can also cross-check your daily carbohydrate using the 'carb flag'. The meals presented below show you how to build a day on the diet using the daily food units on page 71.

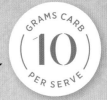

GRAMS CARB
10
PER SERVE

Breakfast

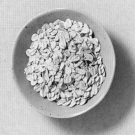 + 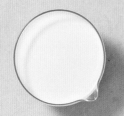 + 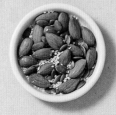 +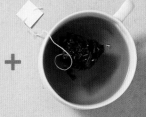

30 g raw oats	180 ml regular milk	30 g nut and seed mix	1 cup of herbal tea
(1 unit Breads, cereals, legumes, starchy veg)	(1 unit Dairy)	(3 units Healthy fats)	(no sugar) ('Free' item)

Lunch

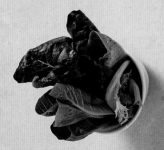 + 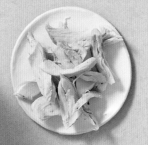 + 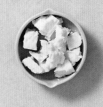 +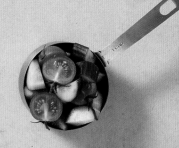

1 cup mixed lettuce
(1 unit Low-carb veg)

100 g cooked pulled chicken
(1 unit Lean meat, fish, poultry, eggs, tofu)

20 g cubed feta cheese
(1 unit Dairy)

1 cup mixed cucumber and tomato
(1 unit Low-carb veg)

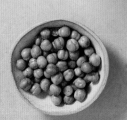 + 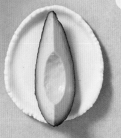 + 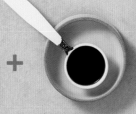 +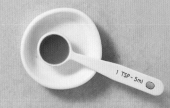

40 g toasted chickpeas
(0.5 unit Breads, cereals, legumes, starchy veg)

40 g avocado
(2 units Healthy fats)

1 tablespoon (20 ml) balsamic vinegar
('Free' item)

1 teaspoon (5 ml) olive oil
(1 unit Healthy fats)

Dinner

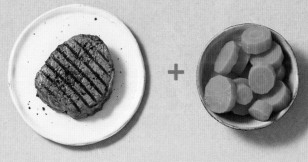

150 g meat, fish, chicken or marinated tofu, grilled to your preference (use a spice rub for flavour) (1.5 units Lean meat, fish, poultry, eggs, tofu)

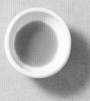

1 cup steamed cooked carrot (1 unit Mod–carb veg)

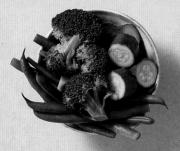 + 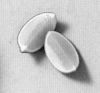 +

1.5 cups mixed steamed veg (zucchini, green beans, broccoli) (1.5 units Low–mod carb veg)

lime juice as desired ('Free' item)

2 teaspoons (10 ml) olive oil for cooking (2 units Healthy fats)

Total units used

1.5 units Breads, cereals, legumes, starchy veg
2.5 units Lean meat
2 units Dairy
4.5 units Low–mod carb veg
8 units Healthy fats

Left over for unit top-ups

1 unit Dairy
2 units Healthy fats
0.5 unit Low–mod carb veg

Unit top-ups

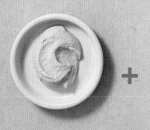 + 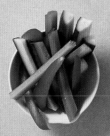 + 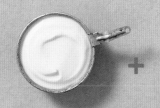 +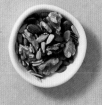

20 g hummus (1 unit Healthy fats)

Sliced cucumber, celery and capsicum sticks (0.5 unit Low–mod carb veg)

100 g yoghurt (no added sugar) (1 unit Dairy)

10 g nut and seed mix (1 unit Healthy fats)

One of the key features of *The CSIRO Low-carb Diabetes Diet & Lifestyle Solution* is to understand how much of these food units you should have at each meal, which is an addition to the regular CSIRO Low-carb Diet – to achieve the best glucose control, you will need a mix of different food groups at each meal, which need to be spread evenly throughout the day.

When adapting your eating routine to improve blood glucose control, we suggest minimising your snacking behaviours, and to use left-over core food units if you are needing something extra in your day as top-ups.

This means having three meals and one unit top-up as a snack in your day. The food units commonly contributing to top-up options will be Dairy, Healthy fats and Low-carb vegetable units. Commonly selected 'core food' snacks would include, for example, 10 grams of nuts or 20 grams of hummus (which equates to 1 Healthy fats unit), or a 100 gram tub of plain yoghurt (1 Dairy unit).

Chat to a dietitian

If you engage in high levels of physical activity, or have irregular meal times for various reasons such as work requirements, talk to your dietitian to determine the best timing of your meals to achieve good glucose control.

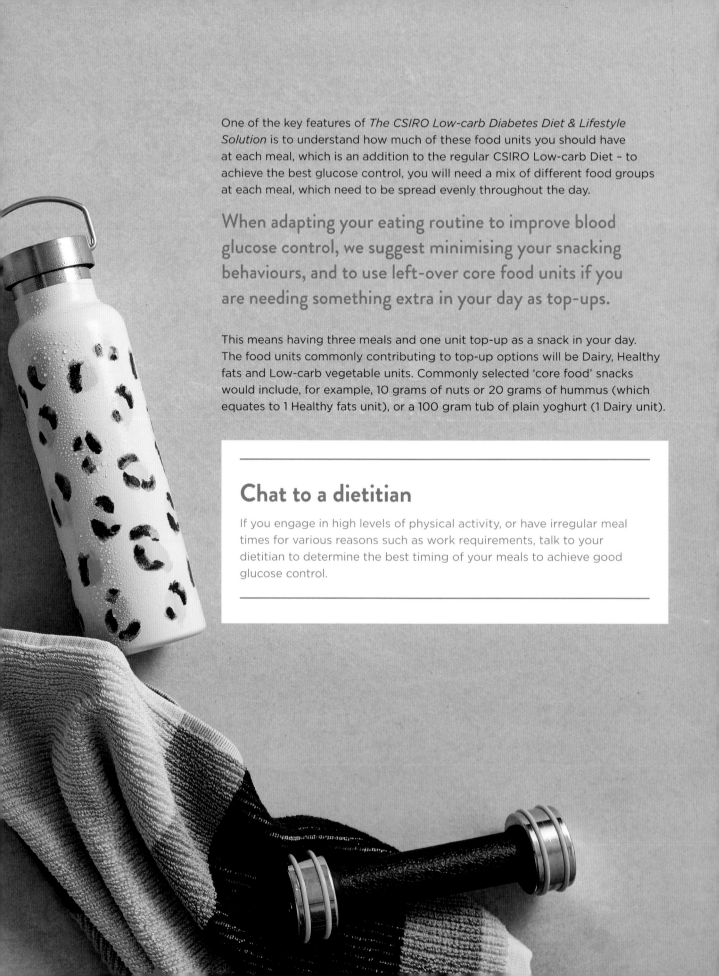

How do I get started on *The CSIRO Low-carb Diabetes Diet & Lifestyle Solution*?

1

Review the background and principles of *The CSIRO Low-carb Diabetes Diet & Lifestyle Solution*

2

Engage and consult your GP and healthcare team before starting on the plan

3

Calculate your individual energy requirements (pages 74–5)

4

Determine the energy level (daily kilojoule intake) that most suits your estimated energy requirements (page 71)

5

For your energy level, refer to the food unit amounts (page 71), then identify the types and quantities of each food group to make up your daily intake of units (pages 79–81)

6

Choose your recipes, using the food units provided per serve to plan your daily and weekly menu – in line with your food unit allowance. Planning ahead saves shopping and preparation time. You can also download food checklists at www.csiro.au/en/Research/Health/CSIRO-diets/Diet-and-recipe-books/CSIRO-Low-Carb-Diet-Book

7

Plan and perform your exercise routine (pages 266–79)

8

Monitor your progress and successes in close consultation with your professional healthcare team.

Meal plans   Week 1

WEEKS 1–6

6000 KJ/50 G CARBOHYDRATES PER DAY

THE FOLLOWING WEEKLY MEAL PLANS SHOW HOW YOU CAN ENJOY YOUR DAILY INTAKE OF UNITS WHILE FOLLOWING THE CSIRO LOW-CARB DIABETES DIET & LIFESTYLE SOLUTION.

Weeks 1–6 are based on the daily 6000 kJ template providing up to 50 grams of carbohydrate (see page 71). The meal plans show you how to incorporate the recipes into your daily menu to achieve the total food units for your given energy level while maintaining good nutrition quality.

In order for you to enjoy a variety of food options across the day, each recipe does not contain the exact same number of units. Therefore, when you are planning your weekly menu, **it is important to pay attention to the individual food units for each recipe, to ensure you meet the correct total for each day.**

Sometimes, if the recipes you have selected do not provide your total amount of daily food units required, you will need to use the remaining units as 'top ups' to ensure you meet your daily total.

This top-up approach also allows you to achieve your total daily food unit allowances if you are following a weekly meal plan with a higher energy level (see page 71).

	MONDAY	TUESDAY
Breakfast	Baked Stuffed Mushrooms (p 158) • 0.5 Breads, cereals, legumes, starchy vegetables • 1 Dairy • 1 Low-carb veg • 2 Healthy fats	Grilled haloumi and vegetables: Grill 20 g haloumi + 2 cups mixed spinach, mushroom, asparagus and tomato + 1 tsp garlic paste + 40 g drained tinned chickpeas. Top with 20 g avocado + 20 g hummus • 0.5 Breads, cereals, legumes, starchy vegetables • 1 Dairy • 2 Low-carb veg • 2 Healthy fats
Lunch	Hearty Tuna Couscous Salad (p 164) • 1 Breads, cereals, legumes, starchy vegetables • 1 Dairy • 1 Lean meat, fish, poultry, eggs, tofu • 2 Low-carb veg • 1 Moderate-carb veg • 3 Healthy fats UNIT TOP-UP 20 g cheddar cheese 20 g raw mixed nuts • 1 Dairy • 2 Healthy fats	Chargrilled Chicken and Mushrooms with Avocado Lentils (p 175) • 1 Breads, cereals, legumes, starchy vegetables • 1 Dairy • 1 Lean meat, fish, poultry, eggs, tofu • 2 Low-carb veg • 3 Healthy fats
Dinner	Roast Beef with Herb Finishing Sauce (p 256) • 1.5 Lean meat, fish, poultry, eggs, tofu • 2 Low-carb veg • 1 Moderate-carb veg • 3 Healthy fats	Tandoori Salmon Tray Bake (p 237) • 1.5 Lean meat, fish, poultry, eggs, tofu • 2 Low-carb veg • 1 Moderate-carb veg • 3 Healthy fats UNIT TOP-UP 100 g plain yoghurt + 20 g raw pistachios and pine nuts • 1 Dairy • 2 Healthy fats
Unit Tally	• 1.5 Breads, cereals, legumes, starchy vegetables • 3 Dairy • 2.5 Lean meat, fish, poultry, eggs, tofu • 5 Low-carb veg • 2 Moderate-carb veg • 10 Healthy fats	• 1.5 Breads, cereals, legumes, starchy vegetables • 3 Dairy • 2.5 Lean meat, fish, poultry, eggs, tofu • 6 Low-carb veg • 1 Moderate-carb veg • 10 Healthy fats

	WEDNESDAY	THURSDAY	FRIDAY	SATURDAY	SUNDAY
Breakfast	15 g low-GI, high-fibre cereal (no added fruit) + 180 ml high-protein milk + 30 g raw mixed nuts and/or seeds + 1 tsp cinnamon (optional) • 0.5 Breads, cereals, legumes, starchy vegetables • 1 Dairy • 3 Healthy fats	Tex-mex Scramble with Chargrilled Corn Salsa (p 137) • 0.5 Breads, cereals, legumes, starchy vegetables • 1 Dairy • 0.5 Lean meat, fish, poultry, eggs, tofu • 2 Low-carb veg • 2 Healthy fats	On-the-run breakfast 1: 150 g high-protein plain yoghurt + 15 g All-Bran Original + 30 g raw mixed nuts and/or seeds • 0.5 Breads, cereals, legumes, starchy vegetables • 1.5 Dairy • 1 Lean meat, fish, poultry, eggs, tofu • 3 Healthy fats **UNIT TOP-UP** Black coffee + 50 ml milk + 8 Brazil nuts • 0.5 Dairy • 3 Healthy fats	Baked Stuffed Mushrooms (p 158) • 0.5 Breads, cereals, legumes, starchy vegetables • 1 Dairy • 1 Low-carb veg • 2 Healthy fats	On-the-run breakfast 2: 2 x rye Cruskits + 3 tsp basil pesto + 20 g cheddar cheese + 1 medium grilled tomato + ½ cup sliced mushrooms • 0.5 Breads, cereals, legumes, starchy vegetables • 1 Dairy • 1 Low-carb veg • 3 Healthy fats
Lunch	Chicken, Cashew and Quinoa Toss (p 194) • 1 Breads, cereals, legumes, starchy vegetables • 1 Dairy • 1 Lean meat, fish, poultry, eggs, tofu • 2 Low-carb veg • 0.5 Moderate-carb veg • 3 Healthy fats	Cajun Tofu with Corn Salsa (p 201) • 1 Breads, cereals, legumes, starchy vegetables • 1 Dairy • 0.5 Lean meat, fish, poultry, eggs, tofu • 2 Low-carb veg • 0.5 Moderate-carb veg • 2 Healthy fats	Salmon Salad With Seasoned Toast (p 168) • 1 Breads, cereals, legumes, starchy vegetables • 1 Dairy • 1 Lean meat, fish, poultry, eggs, tofu • 2 Low-carb veg • 1 Moderate-carb veg • 2 Healthy fats	Chicken and Rice Soup (p 171) • 1 Breads, cereals, legumes, starchy vegetables • 1 Dairy • 1 Lean meat, fish, poultry, eggs, tofu • 2 Low-carb veg • 0.5 Moderate-carb veg • 2 Healthy fats **UNIT TOP-UP** 100 g plain yoghurt + 40 g raw pistachios and pine nuts • 1 Dairy • 4 Healthy fats	Warm Roast Chicken, Veggie and Quinoa Salad (p 197) • 1 Breads, cereals, legumes, starchy vegetables • 1 Dairy • 1 Lean meat, fish, poultry, eggs, tofu • 1 Low-carb veg • 1.5 Moderate-carb veg • 3 Healthy fats
Dinner	Greek Roasted Lamb Cutlets and Veggies (p 260) • 1 Dairy • 1.5 Lean meat, fish, poultry, eggs, tofu • 2 Low-carb veg • 0.5 Moderate-carb veg • 4 Healthy fats	Thai Mushroom Stir-fry with Cauliflower Omelette Rice (p 245) • 1.5 Lean meat, fish, poultry, eggs, tofu • 2 Low-carb veg • 1 Moderate-carb veg • 4 Healthy fats **UNIT TOP-UP** 20 g tasty cheese + 20 g raw almonds + 2 small Lebanese cucumbers • 1 Dairy • 2 Healthy fats • 0.5 Low-carb veg	Smoky Pork and Barbecued Cabbage with Mustard Dressing (p 229) • 1.5 Lean meat, fish, poultry, eggs, tofu • 2 Low-carb veg • 1 Moderate-carb veg • 2 Healthy fats	Beef Fillet Steaks with Korma Vegetables (p 259) • 1.5 Lean meat, fish, poultry, eggs, tofu • 2 Low-carb veg • 1 Moderate-carb veg • 2 Healthy fats	Bocconcini Stuffed Chicken Tray Bake (p 223) • 1 Dairy • 1.5 Lean meat, fish, poultry, eggs, tofu • 2 Low-carb veg • 1 Moderate-carb veg • 4 Healthy fats
Unit Tally	• 1.5 Breads, cereals, legumes, starchy vegetables • 3 Dairy • 2.5 Lean meat, fish, poultry, eggs, tofu • 4 Low-carb veg • 1 Moderate-carb veg • 10 Healthy fats	• 1.5 Breads, cereals, legumes, starchy vegetables • 3 Dairy • 2.5 Lean meat, fish, poultry, eggs, tofu • 6.5 Low-carb veg • 1.5 Moderate-carb veg • 10 Healthy fats	• 1.5 Breads, cereals, legumes, starchy vegetables • 3 Dairy • 2.5 Lean meat, fish, poultry, eggs, tofu • 4 Low-carb veg • 2 Moderate-carb veg • 10 Healthy fats	• 1.5 Breads, cereals, legumes, starchy vegetables • 3 Dairy • 2.5 Lean meat, fish, poultry, eggs, tofu • 5 Low-carb veg • 1.5 Moderate-carb veg • 10 Healthy fats	• 1.5 Breads, cereals, legumes, starchy vegetables • 3 Dairy • 2.5 Lean meat, fish, poultry, eggs, tofu • 4 Low-carb veg • 2.5 Moderate-carb veg • 10 Healthy fats

Pantry shopping list

PANTRY

- mixed unsalted raw nuts and/or seeds: raw almonds (flaked or slivered); Brazil nuts; cashews; macadamias; pecans; pistachios; pine nuts; pumpkin seeds
- tahini and nut butter (cashew, almond or peanut)
- nut butter spread with no added sugar or salt (tahini, cashew or almond)
- untoasted fruit-free muesli
- bread: Herman Brot Lower Carb Bread, seeded bread, wholemeal mountain or pita
- wholegrain crispbreads (9 Grains Vita-Weat, Cruskits, Ryvita) and rice crackers
- low-GI rice
- quinoa
- rolled oats
- wholemeal couscous
- wholemeal spaghetti
- konjac spaghetti
- wholemeal self-raising flour
- artificial sweetener (stevia powder)
- salt-reduced beef/chicken stock
- salt-reduced tomato paste
- baby capers
- tinned tomatoes (diced and chopped)
- tinned red salmon/tuna in spring water
- tinned chickpeas
- tinned lentils
- tinned black beans
- tinned cannellini beans
- tinned red kidney beans
- tinned four-bean mix

SAUCES AND CONDIMENTS

- extra virgin olive oil and olive oil spray
- sesame oil
- sunflower oil
- Dijon mustard
- wholegrain mustard
- balsamic vinegar
- red wine vinegar
- oil-free French dressing
- oil-free Italian dressing
- no added sugar cranberry sauce
- salt-reduced soy sauce
- hoisin sauce
- basil pesto
- passata with basil

HERBS, SPICES AND SEASONING

- garlic
- ginger
- garlic paste
- fresh Italian herb paste
- fresh Thai herb paste
- dried mixed herbs
- lamb dried herbs
- salt-reduced garlic and herb seasoning
- Chinese five-spice powder
- ground cinnamon
- ground ginger
- ground nutmeg
- sweet paprika
- smoked paprika
- sumac
- cocoa powder
- Mexican seasoning
- Cajun spice blend
- harissa spice blend
- peri peri spice blend
- mixed spice
- curry powder
- green curry paste
- korma curry paste
- tandoori paste
- vindaloo curry paste

FRIDGE

- milk
- eggs
- firm tofu
- hummus
- yoghurt
- haloumi
- ricotta
- cottage cheese
- baby bocconcini
- cheddar cheese
- Swiss cheese
- mozzarella
- parmesan
- feta
- Nuttelex olive spread/ olive oil margarine
- cauliflower rice
- zucchini noodles

FREEZER

- frozen broad beans, peeled
- frozen baby peas
- frozen mixed berries

Week 1 meal plan shopping list

QUANTITY	ITEM	QUANTITY	ITEM
	FRUIT		baby spinach and rocket leaf mix
	lemons		English spinach
	limes		tomatoes
			cherry tomatoes
	VEGETABLES		zucchini
	asparagus		
	avocado		**PROTEIN**
	baby bok choy		lean beef fillet steaks
	broccoli		lean beef topside roast
	broccolini		lean chicken breast stir-fry strips
	brussels sprouts		lean chicken tenderloins
	red cabbage		lean French-trimmed lamb cutlets
	red capsicum		lean pork loin steaks
	carrot		skinless, boneless salmon fillet
	cauliflower		
	celery		**OTHER**
	corn		chives
	Lebanese cucumbers		coriander
	baby green beans		dill
	leek		flat-leaf parsley
	cos lettuce		mint
	button mushrooms		oregano
	cup mushrooms		rosemary
	mixed mushrooms (field, portobello, shiitake, button)		
	large field mushrooms		
	red onion		
	spring onions		
	parsnips		
	pumpkin		
	baby radishes		
	baby rocket leaves		
	mixed salad leaves		
	baby spinach leaves		

Week 2

	MONDAY	TUESDAY	WEDNESDAY	THURSDAY	FRIDAY	SATURDAY	SUNDAY
Breakfast	100 g high-protein natural Greek-style yoghurt + 1 tsp passionfruit pulp + 40 g seeds + 10 g flaked almonds + 15 g untoasted muesli	2 x rye Cruskits + 20 g nut butter with no added sugar (cashew, almond or peanut) or 40 g avocado served with 100 g natural Greek-style yoghurt + 30 g seeds	Grilled haloumi and vegetables: Grill 20 g haloumi + 2 cups mixed spinach, mushroom, asparagus and tomato + 1 tsp garlic paste + 40 g drained tinned chickpeas. Top with 20 g avocado + 20 g hummus	2 x 9 Grains Vita-Weat + 4 tsp tahini + 55 g ricotta or cottage cheese **UNIT TOP-UP** 1 small (180 ml) flat white/cappuccino/latte (no sugar or flavours) + 20 g Brazil nuts	Sweet Potato and Feta Omelettes (p 121) **UNIT TOP-UP** 1 small (180 ml) flat white/cappuccino/latte (no sugar or flavours) + 40 g Brazil nuts	Eggplant Subs with Smashed Beans (p 161)	Baked Stuffed Mushrooms (p 158)
Lunch	Creamy Potato Salad with Tuna (p 185)	Cannellini Bean, Chicken and Vegetable Stew (p 179)	Chargrilled Chicken Pasta with Nutty Sauce (p 180)	Tuna, Corn and Capsicum Smash (p 198)	Cajun Tofu with Corn Salsa (p 201)	Chicken Bolognese with Konjac Spaghetti (p 193)	Warm Roast Chicken, Veggie and Quinoa Salad (p 197)
Dinner	Roast Vegetable Frittata (p 242)	One-pan Lemony Chicken and Vegetables (p 217)	Hoisin Barramundi Bowls (p 234) **UNIT TOP-UP** 40 g Black Swan avocado dip + ½ cup sliced cucumber and celery + 20 g cheddar cheese + 20 g raw almonds	Harissa Beef Skewers and Zesty Herb Salad (p 252)	Slow-cooker Chicken Cacciatore with Cauliflower Mash (p 206)	Summer Pesto Prawns with Zucchini Noodles (p 238) **UNIT TOP-UP** 100 g vanilla yoghurt (no added sugar) + 20 g flaked almonds or raw pistachios	Ginger Turkey Stir-fry (p 225) **UNIT TOP-UP** 20 g Black Swan avocado dip + ½ cup sliced cucumber and celery + 20 g cheddar cheese + 20 g raw almonds

Week 2 meal plan shopping list

QUANTITY	ITEM
	FRUIT
	lemons
	limes
	passionfruit
	VEGETABLES
	asparagus
	avocado
	bean sprouts
	Chinese broccoli
	broccoli
	brussels sprouts
	red cabbage
	red capsicum
	carrot
	cauliflower
	celery
	corn
	Lebanese cucumbers
	eggplant
	baby fennel
	baby green beans
	kale
	baby cos lettuce
	iceberg lettuce
	button mushrooms
	field mushrooms
	onion
	red onion
	baby potatoes
	pumpkin
	snow peas
	baby spinach leaves
	English spinach

QUANTITY	ITEM
	sugar snap peas
	baby radishes
	sweet potato
	tomatoes
	mixed baby tomatoes
	roma tomatoes
	zucchini
	PROTEIN
	lean beef fillet
	lean chicken breast fillets
	lean chicken breast stir-fry strips
	lean chicken tenderloins
	lean turkey breast fillet
	skinless, boneless barramundi fillets
	cooked peeled, deveined medium tiger prawns
	OTHER
	basil
	long green chillies
	chives
	coriander
	flat-leaf parsley
	micro herbs (optional)
	mint
	Black Swan avocado dip
	tin sliced bamboo shoots
	pitted green Sicilian olives

Week 3

	MONDAY	TUESDAY	WEDNESDAY	THURSDAY	FRIDAY	SATURDAY	SUNDAY
Breakfast	Sweet Potato and Feta Omelettes (p 121) **UNIT TOP-UP** 20 g raw almonds	Scramble Pita Pockets (p 117)	30 g low-GI, high-fibre cereal (no added fruit) + 180 ml milk + 20 g raw mixed nuts and/or seeds	1 x 30 g sachet porridge + 100 g high-protein plain yoghurt + 30 g raw macadamias	Baked Stuffed Mushrooms (p 158)	1 Hi-Bran Weet-Bix + 100 g vanilla yoghurt (no added sugar) + 40 g raw mixed nuts and/or seeds + 1 tsp cinnamon (optional)	Weet-Bix and Yoghurt Bliss Balls (p 145)
Lunch	Mexican Fish and Black Beans (p 167) + 2 x high-fibre low-GI crispbreads + 2 tsp Nuttelex olive spread	Cajun Tofu with Corn Salsa (p 201) **UNIT TOP-UP** 100 g vanilla yoghurt (no added sugar) + 20 g raw mixed nuts	Quick and easy tofu crispbreads: 3 x Ryvita or 9 Grains Vita-Weat + 20 g hummus + 1 sliced medium tomato + 1 cup baby spinach + 100 g sliced tofu + 20 g avocado + 20 g Swiss or cheddar cheese	Sashimi Salmon with Caper Avocado Dressing (p 189)	Chicken, Cashew and Quinoa Toss (p 194)	Hearty Tuna Couscous Salad (p 164)	Curried Egg Salad with Mountain Bread (p 190)
Dinner	Balsamic Marinated Beef with Tomatoes (p 248)	Thai Mushroom Stir-fry with Cauliflower Omelette Rice (p 245)	Tandoori Salmon Tray Bake (p 237) **UNIT TOP-UP** 20 g Black Swan avocado dip + ½ cup sliced cucumber and celery + 20 g cheddar cheese + 20 g raw almonds	Chargrilled Chicken with Celery Salad (p 205) **UNIT TOP-UP** 20 g cheddar cheese + 10 g raw cashews	Greek Roasted Lamb Cutlets and Veggies (p 260) + 10 g raw cashews	Roast Vegetable Frittata (p 242)	Chilli Squid with Nutty Cucumber Salad (p 233) **UNIT TOP-UP** 20 g raw cashews + 20 g raw almonds

Week 3 meal plan shopping list

QUANTITY	ITEM	QUANTITY	ITEM
	FRUIT		cherry tomatoes
	lemons		roma tomatoes
	limes		zucchini
	VEGETABLES		**PROTEIN**
	asparagus		lean beef fillet steaks
	avocado		lean chicken breast fillets
	baby bok choy		lean chicken breast stir-fry strips
	broccoli florets		lean French-trimmed lamb cutlets
	red capsicum		skinless, boneless flathead fillets
	cauliflower		skinless, boneless salmon fillets
	celery		sashimi-grade salmon
	corn		cleaned fresh squid hoods
	Lebanese cucumbers		
	baby fennel		**OTHER**
	baby green beans		basil
	cos lettuce		long red chillies
	baby cos lettuce		chives
	baby gem lettuce		coriander
	cup mushrooms		flat-leaf parsley
	mixed mushrooms (field, portobello, shiitake, button)		mint
	large field mushrooms		
	pumpkin		micro herbs (optional)
	baby radishes		Black Swan avocado dip
	baby rocket leaves		
	mixed salad leaves		
	baby spinach leave		
	baby spinach and rocket leaf mix		
	English spinach		
	red onion		
	baby yellow squash		
	sweet potato		

Week 4

	MONDAY	TUESDAY	WEDNESDAY	THURSDAY	FRIDAY	SATURDAY	SUNDAY
Breakfast	Frozen Cereal and Yoghurt Discs (p 138)	Oat and Almond Caramel Shake (p 141)	Scramble Pita Pockets (p 117) **UNIT TOP-UP** 100 g plain yoghurt + 30 g raw mixed nuts and/or seeds	Spinach and Cheddar Bakes (p 130)	Individual Fruit Toast Puddings (p 134)	Lentil Breakfast Bowl (p 146)	Poached Eggs with Veggies and Pesto Parmesan Yoghurt (p 150) **UNIT TOP-UP** 2 x 9 Grains Vita-Weats + 2 tsp nut butter with no added sugar (almond, cashew or macadamia)
Lunch	Turkey salad: 100 g turkey + 20 g low-fat cheese + 1 tsp cranberry sauce (no added sugar) + 1 cup salad leaves + 40 g avocado + 1 slice Herman Brot Lower Carb bread **UNIT TOP-UP** 20 g Black Swan avocado dip + 150 g low-carb veg + 20 g cheddar cheese + 20 g raw almonds	Curried Egg Salad with Mountain Bread (p 190)	Chicken and Rice Soup (p 171)	Chicken, pesto and avocado grill: 1 slice Herman Brot Lower Carb bread + 1 Tbsp basil pesto + 50 g chicken breast + ½ cup baby spinach + 20 g Swiss cheese + 20 g avocado. Grill until cheese is slightly melted **UNIT TOP-UP** 30 g dry-roasted cashews	Quick tuna salad bowl: Add 50 g drained tinned tuna to 40 g drained tinned chickpeas, blend together with 1 Tbsp lemon juice and 2 tsp olive oil. Mix 2 cups salad leaves with ½ cup grated carrot + ½ cup sliced cucumber. Add tuna mixture. Top with 40 g parmesan + 20 g chopped pecans	Chicken Bolognese with Konjac Spaghetti (p 193)	Mexican Fish and Black Beans (p 167)
Dinner	Slow-cooker Chicken Cacciatore with Cauliflower Mash (p 206)	Roast Thai Pork and Broccoli (p 226) **UNIT TOP-UP** 20 g Black Swan avocado dip + 150 g low-carb veg + 20 g cheddar cheese + 20 g raw almonds	Tandoori Salmon Tray Bake (p 237)	Vindaloo Lamb and Eggplant with Raita (p 263)	Five-spice Beef Stir-fry and Hoisin Greens (p 255) **UNIT TOP-UP** 20 g raw macadamias	Roast Vegetable Frittata (p 242) **UNIT TOP-UP** 30 g raw cashews	Bocconcini Stuffed Chicken Tray Bake (p 223)

Week 4 meal plan shopping list

QUANTITY	ITEM
	FRUIT
	lemons
	limes
	VEGETABLES
	artichoke
	asparagus
	avocado
	broccoli
	broccolini
	brussels sprouts
	red capsicum
	cauliflower
	celery
	Lebanese cucumbers
	eggplant
	baby fennel
	baby green beans
	leek
	button mushrooms
	cup mushrooms
	red onion
	pumpkin
	baby rocket leaves
	mixed salad leaves
	superleaf salad mix
	snow peas
	baby spinach leaves
	tomatoes
	roma tomatoes
	watercress
	zucchini

QUANTITY	ITEM
	PROTEIN
	lean rump steak
	lean chicken breast fillets
	lean chicken tenderloins
	lean lamb backstraps
	lean pork fillets
	roast turkey
	skinless, boneless salmon fillets
	skinless, boneless flathead fillets
	OTHER
	basil
	chives
	coriander
	flat-leaf parsley
	mint
	Black Swan avocado dip
	pitted green Sicilian olives
	diet caramel topping

Week 5

	MONDAY	TUESDAY	WEDNESDAY	THURSDAY	FRIDAY	SATURDAY	SUNDAY
Breakfast	Baked Stuffed Mushrooms (p 158)	2 x 9 Grains Vita-Weat + 1 Tbsp tahini + 55 g ricotta or cottage cheese **UNIT TOP-UP** 180 ml full-cream milk (can be added to coffee or tea — no added sugar or flavours)	Bruschetta with Bocconcini and Pecans (p 128)	Scramble Pita Pockets (p 117)	15 g high-fibre cereal (no added fruit or sugar) + 100 g high-protein Greek-style yoghurt + 40 g raw mixed nuts and/or seeds + 1 tsp cinnamon (optional)	100 g high-protein Greek-style yoghurt + 1 tsp passionfruit pulp + 40 g seeds + 10 g flaked almonds + 15 g untoasted muesli	Grilled haloumi and vegetables: Grill 40 g haloumi + 1 cup mixed spinach, mushroom, asparagus and tomato + 1 tsp garlic paste + 40 g drained tinned chickpeas + 40 g avocado + 20 g hummus
Lunch	Hearty Tuna Couscous Salad (p 164) **UNIT TOP-UP** 20 g raw mixed nuts	Chargrilled Chicken Pasta with Nutty Sauce (p 180)	Curried Egg Salad with Mountain Bread (p 190) **UNIT TOP-UP** 3 medium celery sticks + 20 g tahini or nut butter with no added sugar (cashew or almond)	Tuna, avocado and bean salad: Mix 50 g drained tinned tuna + 40 g drained tinned chickpeas + 80 g diced avocado + 2 tsp hummus mixed with 2 tsp lemon juice + 2 cups salad leaves + 20 g crumbled feta	Chicken, Cashew and Quinoa Toss (p 194)	Creamy Potato Salad with Tuna (p 185)	Rosemary Potato and Chicken Bake (p 186)
Dinner	Roast Beef with Herb Finishing Sauce (p 256)	Summer Pesto Prawns with Zucchini Noodles (p 238)	Roasted Meatballs with Tomato Olive Sauce (p 222)	Warm Chicken and Bean Sprout Salad (p 213) **UNIT TOP-UP** 100 g vanilla yoghurt (no added sugar) + 10 g slivered almonds + ½ tsp ground nutmeg (optional)	Roast Thai Pork and Broccoli (p 226) **UNIT TOP-UP** ½ cup sliced low-carb veg + 55 g ricotta or cottage cheese	Roast Vegetable Frittata (p 242)	Tandoori Salmon Tray Bake (p 237) **UNIT TOP-UP** ½ cup sliced low-carb veg + 40 g hummus

Week 5 meal plan shopping list

QUANTITY	ITEM
	FRUIT
	lemons
	passionfruit
	VEGETABLES
	asparagus
	avocado
	bean sprouts
	broccoli
	broccolini
	Chinese cabbage (wombok)
	cauliflower
	celery
	Lebanese cucumbers
	baby fennel
	baby green beans
	baby cos lettuce
	cup mushrooms
	large field mushrooms
	red onion
	spring onions
	parsnips
	potatoes
	baby potatoes
	pumpkin
	baby radishes
	baby rocket leaves
	mixed salad leaves
	baby spinach leaves
	baby spinach and rocket leaf mix
	tomatoes

QUANTITY	ITEM
	mixed baby tomatoes
	roma tomatoes
	zucchini
	sliced low-carb veg
	PROTEIN
	lean beef topside roast
	lean chicken breast fillets
	lean chicken breast stir-fry strips
	skinless, boneless salmon fillets
	cooked peeled, deveined medium tiger prawns
	Gruyere cheese
	OTHER
	basil
	chives
	flat-leaf parsley
	mint
	oregano
	rosemary
	pitted small Kalamata olives
	ciabatta

Week 6

	MONDAY	TUESDAY	WEDNESDAY	THURSDAY	FRIDAY	SATURDAY	SUNDAY
Breakfast	2 x rye Cruskits + 20 g nut butter with no added sugar (cashew, almond or peanut) or 40 g avocado. Side of 100 g natural Greek-style yoghurt + 30 g seeds	Scramble Pita Pockets (p 117) **UNIT TOP-UP** 100 g vanilla yoghurt (no added sugar) + 20 g raw mixed nuts	Eggplant Subs with Smashed Beans (p 161)	On-the-run breakfast 1: 150 g high-protein plain yoghurt + 15 g All-Bran Original + 30 g raw mixed nuts and/or seeds **UNIT TOP-UP** Black coffee + 90 ml milk (no sugar) + 6 x Brazil nuts	Roasted Greens with Eggs (p 118)	Couscous Scramble (p 155)	Baked Stuffed Mushrooms (p 158)
Lunch	Cannellini Bean, Chicken and Vegetable Stew (p 179)	Cajun Tofu with Corn Salsa (p 201)	Chicken Bolognese with Konjac Spaghetti (p 193)	Salmon Salad with Seasoned Toast (p 168)	Chicken salad: Mix 50 g roast chicken + 80 g drained tinned chickpeas + 20 g grated cheddar cheese + 3 tsp olive oil + 2 tsp lime or lemon juice + 2 cups salad leaves + ½ cup sliced tomato and red onion + 30 g pumpkin seeds	Mexican Fish and Black Beans (p 167)	Chicken, Cashew and Quinoa Toss (p 194)
Dinner	One-pan Lemony Chicken and Vegetables (p 217)	Thai Mushroom Stir-fry with Cauliflower Omelette Rice (p 245)	Summer Pesto Prawns with Zucchini Noodles (p 238) **UNIT TOP-UP** 100 g vanilla yoghurt (no added sugar) + 20 g flaked almonds or raw pistachios	Smoky Pork and Barbecued Cabbage with Mustard Dressing (p 229)	Vindaloo Lamb and Eggplant with Raita (p 263)	Steam-roasted Chicken with Fresh Tomato Pesto (p 221) **UNIT TOP-UP** 20 g dry-roasted cashews	Greek Roasted Lamb Cutlets and Veggies (p 260) + 10 g raw cashews

Week 6 meal plan shopping list

QUANTITY	ITEM
	FRUIT
	lemons
	limes
	VEGETABLES
	asparagus
	avocado
	baby bok choy
	broccoli
	red cabbage
	red capsicum
	carrot
	cauliflower
	celery
	corn
	Lebanese cucumbers
	eggplant
	baby green beans
	cos lettuce
	mixed mushrooms (field, portobello, shiitake, button)
	field mushrooms
	onion
	red onion
	spring onions
	pumpkin
	baby radishes
	baby rocket leaves
	mixed salad leaves
	superleaf salad mix
	baby spinach leaves
	baby spinach and rocket leaf mix
	English spinach
	tomatoes

QUANTITY	ITEM
	baby tomatoes
	cherry tomatoes
	zucchini
	PROTEIN
	lean chicken breast fillets
	lean chicken breast stir-fry strips
	roast chicken
	lean lamb backstraps
	lean French-trimmed lamb cutlets
	skinless, boneless flathead fillets
	cooked peeled, deveined medium tiger prawns
	OTHER
	basil
	coriander
	flat-leaf parsley
	mint

Meal plans

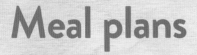

WEEKS 7–12

6500 KJ/70 G CARBOHYDRATES PER DAY

The meal plans for Weeks 7–12 show you some easy ways of adding 20 grams of carbohydrate extras (see page 93), using a similar approach to the unit top-ups to provide 70 grams of carbohydrate per day. Weeks 7–12 are also designed to provide an additional 500 kJ daily. Note that the carb extras are optional, and if you are managing well without them, you can simply repeat Weeks 1–6.

Week 7

	MONDAY	TUESDAY	WEDNESDAY	THURSDAY	FRIDAY	SATURDAY	SUNDAY
Breakfast	Baked Stuffed Mushrooms (p 158)	Grilled haloumi and vegetables: Grill 20 g haloumi + 2 cups mixed spinach, mushroom, asparagus and tomato + 1 tsp garlic paste + 40 g drained tinned chickpeas + 20 g avocado + 20 g hummus **Carb Extra** 2 x 9 Grains Vita-Weats	15 g low-GI, high-fibre cereal (no added fruit) + 180 ml high-protein milk + 30 g raw mixed nuts and/or seeds + 1 tsp cinnamon (optional)	Tex-mex Scramble with Chargrilled Corn Salsa (p 137) **Carb Extra** 75 g natural Greek-style yoghurt + 60 g fresh or frozen mixed berries	On-the-run breakfast 1: 100 g plain high-protein yoghurt + 15 g All-Bran Original + 30 g raw mixed nuts and/or seeds **UNIT TOP-UP** Black coffee + 50 ml milk (no sugar) + 6 x Brazil nuts	Curried Frying-pan Eggs (p 154) **Carb Extra** 75 g natural Greek-style yoghurt + 60 g fresh or frozen mixed berries	On-the-run breakfast 2: 2 x rye Cruskits + 3 tsp basil pesto + 20 g cheddar cheese + 1 medium grilled tomato + ½ cup sliced mushrooms
Lunch	Hearty Tuna Cous-cous Salad (p 164) **UNIT TOP-UP** 20 g mixed raw nuts **Carb Extra** 20 g dried fruit	Chargrilled Chicken and Mushrooms with Avocado Lentils (p 175)	Chicken, Cashew and Quinoa Toss (p 194)	Cajun Tofu with Corn Salsa (p 201)	Salmon Salad with Seasoned Toast (p 168) **Carb Extra** 2 kiwifruit	Chicken and Rice Soup (p 171) **UNIT TOP-UP** 100 g plain yoghurt + 40 g raw pistachios and pine nuts	Warm Roast Chicken, Veggie and Quinoa Salad (p 197)
Dinner	Roast Beef with Herb Finishing Sauce (p 256)	Tandoori Salmon Tray Bake (p 237) **UNIT TOP-UP** 100 g plain yoghurt + 20 g raw pistachios and pine nuts **Carb Extra** 60 g blueberries	Greek Roasted Lamb Cutlets and Veggies (p 260) **Carb Extra** Add 100 g roasted sweet potato	Thai Mushroom Stir-fry with Cauliflower Omelette Rice (p 245) **UNIT TOP-UP** 20 g cheddar cheese + 20 g raw almonds + 2 small Lebanese cucumbers	Smoky Pork and Barbecued Cabbage with Mustard Dressing (p 229)	Beef Fillet Steaks with Korma Vegetables (p 259)	Bocconcini Stuffed Chicken Tray Bake (p 223) **Carb Extra** 1 navel orange

Week 7 meal plan shopping list

QUANTITY	ITEM	QUANTITY	ITEM
	FRUIT		parsnips
	blueberries		pumpkin
	mixed dried fruit		baby radishes
	kiwifruit		baby rocket leaves
	lemons		mixed salad leaves
	limes		spinach
	navel oranges		baby spinach leaves
			baby spinach and rocket leaf mix
	VEGETABLES		English spinach
	asparagus		sweet potato
	avocado		tomatoes
	baby bok choy		cherry tomatoes
	whole peeled broad beans		zucchini
	broccoli		
	broccolini		**PROTEIN**
	brussels sprouts		lean beef fillet steaks
	red cabbage		lean beef topside roast
	red capsicum		lean chicken breast fillets
	carrot		lean chicken breast stir-fry strips
	cauliflower		lean chicken tenderloins
	celery		lean French-trimmed lamb cutlets
	corn		lean pork loin steaks
	fresh corn kernels		skinless, boneless salmon fillets
	Lebanese cucumbers		
	baby green beans		**OTHER**
	leek		chives
	cos lettuce		coriander
	cup mushrooms		dill
	mixed mushrooms (field, portobello, shiitake, button)		flat-leaf parsley
	large field mushrooms		mint
	button mushrooms		oregano
	red onion		rosemary
	spring onions		

Week 8

	MONDAY	TUESDAY	WEDNESDAY	THURSDAY	FRIDAY	SATURDAY	SUNDAY
Breakfast	100 g high-protein Greek-style yoghurt + 1 tsp passionfruit pulp + 40 g seed mix + 10 g flaked almonds + 15 g untoasted fruit-free muesli **Carb Extra** Add an extra 15 g untoasted fruit-free muesli	2 x rye Cruskits + 20 g nut butter with no added sugar (cashew, almond or peanut) or 40 g avocado. Side of 100 g natural Greek-style yoghurt + 30 g seeds	Grilled haloumi and vegetables: Grill 20 g haloumi + 2 cups mixed spinach, mushroom, asparagus and tomato + 1 tsp garlic paste + 40 g drained tinned chickpeas + 20 g avocado + 20 g hummus	2 x 9 Grains Vita-Weats + 4 tsp tahini + 55 g ricotta or cottage cheese **UNIT TOP-UP** 1 small (180 ml) flat white/cappuccino/latte (no sugar or flavours) + 20 g Brazil nuts	Sweet Potato and Feta Omelettes (p 121) **UNIT TOP-UP** 1 small (180 ml) flat white/cappuccino/latte (no sugar or flavours) + 40 g Brazil nuts	Eggplant Subs with Smashed Beans (p 161) **Carb Extra** 1 x slice seeded low-carb bread	Baked Stuffed Mushrooms (p 158) **Carb Extra** 1 medium just-ripe banana
Lunch	Creamy Potato Salad with Tuna (p 185)	Cannellini Bean, Chicken and Vegetable Stew (p 179)	Chargrilled Chicken Pasta with Nutty Sauce (p 180)	Tuna, Corn and Capsicum Smash (p 198)	Cajun Tofu with Corn Salsa (p 201)	Chicken Bolognese with Konjac Spaghetti (p 193)	Warm Roast Chicken, Veggie and Quinoa Salad (p 197)
Dinner	Roast Vegetable Frittata (p 242) **Carb Extra** 2 x 9 Grains Vita-Weats + vegemite	One-pan Lemony Chicken and Vegetables (p 217) **Carb Extra** Add 100 g roasted sweet potato	Hoisin Barramundi Bowls (p 234) **UNIT TOP-UP** 40 g Black Swan avocado dip + ½ cup sliced cucumber and celery + 20 g cheddar cheese + 20 g raw almonds **Carb Extra** 10 x wholegrain rice crackers	Harissa Beef Skewers and Zesty Herb Salad (p 252) **Carb Extra** Add 120 g cooked peas to the salad	Slow-cooker Chicken Cacciatore with Cauliflower Mash (p 206) **Carb Extra** 75 g natural Greek-style yoghurt + 60 g fresh or frozen mixed berries	Summer Pesto Prawns with Zucchini Noodles (p 238) **UNIT TOP-UP** 100 g vanilla yoghurt (no added sugar) + 20 g flaked almonds or raw pistachios	Ginger Turkey Stir-fry (p 225) **UNIT TOP-UP** 20 g Black Swan avocado dip + ½ cup sliced cucumber and celery + 20 g cheddar cheese + 20 g raw almonds

Week 8 meal plan shopping list

QUANTITY	ITEM
	FRUIT
	bananas
	lemons
	limes
	passionfruit
	VEGETABLES
	avocado
	asparagus
	bean sprouts
	broccoli
	Chinese broccoli
	brussels sprouts
	red cabbage
	red capsicum
	carrot
	cauliflower
	celery
	Lebanese cucumbers
	corn
	eggplant
	baby fennel
	baby green beans
	long green chillies
	baby cos lettuce
	iceberg lettuce
	mushrooms
	button mushrooms
	field mushrooms
	onion
	red onion
	baby potatoes
	pumpkin
	baby peas (frozen)

QUANTITY	ITEM
	baby radishes
	spinach
	baby spinach leaves
	English spinach
	sweet potato
	tomatoes
	roma tomatoes
	mixed baby tomatoes
	zucchini
	PROTEIN
	lean beef fillet
	lean chicken breast fillets
	lean chicken breast stir-fry strips
	cooked peeled, deveined medium tiger prawns
	OTHER
	basil
	chives
	coriander
	flat-leaf parsley
	mint
	Black Swan avocado dip
	Vegemite
	tin sliced bamboo shoots

Week 9

	MONDAY	TUESDAY	WEDNESDAY	THURSDAY	FRIDAY	SATURDAY	SUNDAY
Breakfast	Sweet Potato and Feta Omelettes (p 121) **UNIT TOP-UP** 20 g raw almonds	Scramble Pita Pockets (p 117) **Carb Extra** 75 g natural Greek-style yoghurt + 100 g strawberries	30 g low-GI, high-fibre cereal (no added fruit) + 180 ml milk + 20 g raw mixed nuts and/or seeds	1 x 30 g sachet porridge (no added sugar) + 100 g high-protein plain yoghurt + 30 g raw macadamias	Baked Stuffed Mushrooms (p 158) **Carb Extra** 1 x slice seeded low-carb bread	1 Hi-Bran Weet-Bix + 100 g vanilla yoghurt (no added sugar) + 40 g raw mixed nuts and/or seeds + 1 tsp cinnamon (optional)	Weet-Bix and Yoghurt Bliss Balls (p 145)
Lunch	Mexican Fish and Black Beans (p 167) + 2 x high-fibre low-GI crispbreads + 2 tsp Nuttelex olive spread	Cajun Tofu with Corn Salsa (p 201) **UNIT TOP-UP** 100 g vanilla yoghurt (no added sugar) + 20 g raw mixed nuts and/or seeds	Quick and easy tofu crispbreads: 3 x Ryvita or 9 Grains Vita-Weats + 20 g hummus + 1 sliced medium tomato + 1 cup baby spinach + 100 g sliced tofu + 20 g avocado + 20 g Swiss or cheddar cheese	Sashimi Salmon with Caper Avocado Dressing (p 189)	Chicken, Cashew and Quinoa Toss (p 194)	Hearty Tuna Couscous Salad (p 164)	Curried Egg Salad with Mountain Bread (p 190) **Carb Extra** Add 80 g drained tinned four-bean mix
Dinner	Balsamic Marinated Beef with Tomatoes (p 248) **Carb Extra** Add 100 g roasted sweet potato	Thai Mushroom Stir-fry with Cauliflower Omelette Rice (p 245)	Tandoori Salmon Tray Bake (p 237) **UNIT TOP-UP** 20 g Black Swan avocado dip + ½ cup sliced cucumber and celery + 20 g cheddar cheese + 20 g raw almonds **Carb Extra** 200 g strawberries	Chargrilled Chicken with Celery Salad (p 205) **UNIT TOP-UP** 20 g cheddar cheese + 10 g raw cashews **Carb Extra** 5 x wholegrain rice crackers	Greek Roasted Lamb Cutlets and Veggies (p 260) + 10 g raw cashews	Roast Vegetable Frittata (p 242) **Carb Extra** 1 x slice seeded low-carb bread	Chilli Squid with Nutty Cucumber Salad (p 233) **UNIT TOP-UP** 20 g raw cashews + 20 g raw almonds

Week 9 meal plan shopping list

QUANTITY	ITEM
	FRUIT
	lemons
	limes
	strawberries
	VEGETABLES
	asparagus
	avocado
	baby bok choy
	broccoli
	red capsicum
	cauliflower
	celery
	corn
	Lebanese cucumbers
	baby fennel
	baby green beans
	cos lettuce
	baby gem lettuce
	cup mushrooms
	field mushrooms
	mixed mushrooms (field, portobello, shiitake, button)
	red onion
	pumpkin
	baby radishes
	baby rocket leaves
	mixed salad leaves
	baby spinach leaves
	baby spinach and rocket leaf mix
	English spinach
	baby yellow squash
	sweet potato
	tomatoes

QUANTITY	ITEM
	cherry tomatoes
	roma tomatoes
	zucchini
	PROTEIN
	lean beef fillet steaks
	lean chicken breast stir-fry strips
	lean French-trimmed lamb cutlets
	skinless, boneless flathead fillets
	skinless, boneless salmon fillets
	sashimi-grade salmon
	cleaned fresh squid hoods
	OTHER
	basil
	long red chillies
	chives
	coriander
	dill
	flat-leaf parsley
	mint
	Black Swan avocado dip

Week 10

	MONDAY	TUESDAY	WEDNESDAY	THURSDAY	FRIDAY	SATURDAY	SUNDAY
Breakfast	Frozen Cereal and Yoghurt Discs (p 138)	Oat and Almond Caramel Shake (p 141)	Scramble Pita Pockets (p 117) **UNIT TOP-UP** 100 g plain yoghurt + 30 g mixed nuts and seeds	Spinach and Cheddar Bakes (p 130) **Carb Extra** 2 kiwifruit	Individual Fruit Toast Puddings (p 134)	Lentil Breakfast Bowl (p 146) **Carb Extra** 1 small lady finger banana	Poached Eggs with Veggies and Pesto Parmesan Yoghurt (p 150) **UNIT TOP-UP** 2 x 9 Grains Vita-Weats + 2 tsp nut butter with no added sugar (almond, cashew or macadamia)
Lunch	Turkey salad: 100 g roast turkey + 20 g low-fat cheese + 1 tsp cranberry sauce (no added sugar) + 1 cup salad leaves + 40 g sliced avocado on 1 slice Herman Brot Lower Carb bread **UNIT TOP-UP** 20 g Black Swan avocado dip + 150 g sliced low-carb veg + 20 g cheddar cheese + 20 g raw almonds	Curried Egg Salad with Mountain Bread (p 190) **Carb Extra** Add 80 g drained tinned chickpeas + 2 tsp lemon juice	Chicken and Rice Soup (p 171)	Chicken, pesto and avocado open grill: 1 x slice Herman Brot Lower Carb bread + 1 tbsp basil pesto + 50 g chicken breast + ½ cup baby spinach + 20 g Swiss cheese + 20 g sliced avocado. Grill until cheese is slightly melted **UNIT TOP-UP** 30 g roasted unsalted cashews	Quick tuna salad bowl: Add 50 g drained tinned tuna to 40 g drained tinned chickpeas, mix together with 1 tbsp lemon juice and 2 tsp olive oil. Mix 2 cups salad leaves with ½ cup grated carrot + ½ cup sliced cucumber. Add tuna mixture + top with 40 g shaved parmesan + 20 g chopped pecans	Chicken Bolognese with Konjac Spaghetti (p 193)	Mexican Fish and Black Beans (p 167)
Dinner	Slow-cooker Chicken Cacciatore with Cauliflower Mash (p 206) **Carb Extra** 1 navel orange	Roast Thai Pork and Broccoli (p 226) **UNIT TOP-UP** 20 g Black Swan avocado dip + 150 g sliced low-carb veg + 20 g cheddar cheese + 20 g raw almonds	Tandoori Salmon Tray Bake (p 237) **Carb Extra** 75 g natural Greek-style yoghurt + 60 g fresh or frozen mixed berries	Vindaloo Lamb and Eggplant Raita (p 263)	Five-spice Beef Stir-fry and Hoisin Greens (p 255) **UNIT TOP-UP** 20 g raw macadamias **Carb Extra** 2 small dried figs	Roast Vegetable Frittata (p 242) **UNIT TOP-UP** 30 g raw cashews	Bocconcini Stuffed Chicken Tray Bake (p 223) **Carb Extra** 50 g chopped apple + 50 g chopped pear

Week 10 meal plan shopping list

QUANTITY	ITEM
	FRUIT
	apples
	lady finger bananas
	small dried figs
	kiwifruit
	lemons
	limes
	navel oranges
	pears
	VEGETABLES
	artichoke
	asparagus
	avocado
	broccoli
	red capsicum
	carrot
	cauliflower
	celery
	Lebanese cucumbers
	eggplant
	baby fennel
	baby green beans
	leek
	button mushrooms
	cup mushrooms
	onion
	red onion
	baby peas (frozen)
	pumpkin
	baby rocket leaves
	superleaf salad mix
	snow peas
	baby spinach leaves

QUANTITY	ITEM
	tomatoes
	roma tomatoes
	watercress
	zucchini
	PROTEIN
	lean rump steak
	lean chicken breast fillets
	lean chicken tenderloins
	lean lamb backstraps
	lean pork fillet
	roast turkey
	skinless, boneless flathead fillets
	skinless, boneless salmon fillets
	OTHER
	basil
	chives
	coriander
	flat-leaf parsley
	mint
	Black Swan avocado dip
	fruit bread
	pitted green Sicilian olives
	diet caramel topping

Week 11

	MONDAY	TUESDAY	WEDNESDAY	THURSDAY	FRIDAY	SATURDAY	SUNDAY
Breakfast	Baked Stuffed Mushrooms (p 158) **Carb Extra** Add 1 x slice seeded low-carb bread	2 x 9 Grains Vita-Weats + 4 tsp tahini + 55 g ricotta or cottage cheese **UNIT TOP-UP** 180 ml full-cream milk (can be added to coffee or tea — no added sugar or flavours)	Bruschetta with Bocconcini and Pecans (p 128)	Scramble Pita Pockets (p 117) **Carb Extra** 75 g natural Greek-style yoghurt + 60 g fresh or frozen mixed berries	15 g high-fibre cereal (no added fruit or sugar) + 100 g natural Greek-style yoghurt + 40 g raw mixed nuts and/or seeds + 1 tsp cinnamon (optional)	100 g high-protein Greek-style yoghurt + 1 tsp passionfruit pulp + 40 g seeds + 10 g flaked almonds + 15 g untoasted muesli	Grilled haloumi and vegetables: 40 g grilled haloumi + 1 cup mixed spinach, mushroom, asparagus and tomato + 1 tsp garlic paste + 40 g drained tinned chickpeas + 40 g avocado + 20 g hummus **Carb Extra** Add 40 g chickpeas + 40 g corn kernels
Lunch	Hearty Tuna Couscous Salad (p 164) **UNIT TOP-UP** 20 g raw mixed nuts	Chargrilled Chicken Pasta with Nutty Sauce (p 180)	Curried Egg Salad with Mountain Bread (p 190) **UNIT TOP-UP** 3 medium celery sticks + 20 g tahini **Carb Extra** 10 x wholegrain rice crackers	Tuna, avocado and bean salad: Mix 50 g drained tinned tuna + 40 g drained tinned chickpeas + 80 g avocado + 2 tsp hummus + 2 tsp lemon juice + 2 cups salad leaves + 20 g crumbled feta	Chicken, Cashew and Quinoa Toss (p 194)	Creamy Potato Salad with Tuna (p 185)	Rosemary Potato and Chicken Bake (p 186)
Dinner	Roast Beef with Herb Finishing Sauce (p 256)	Summer Pesto Prawns with Zucchini Noodles (p 238) **Carb Extra** Add 100 g drained cannellini beans	Roasted Meatballs with Tomato Olive Sauce (p 222)	Warm Chicken and Bean Sprout Salad (p 213) **UNIT TOP-UP** 100 g vanilla yoghurt (no added sugar) + 10 g slivered almonds + ½ tsp ground nutmeg (optional)	Roast Thai Pork and Broccoli (p 226) **UNIT TOP-UP** ½ cup sliced low-carb veg + 55 g ricotta or cottage cheese **Carb Extra** 4 dried dates	Roast Vegetable Frittata (p 242) **Carb Extra** 200 g strawberries	Tandoori Salmon Tray Bake (p 237) **UNIT TOP-UP** ½ cup sliced low-carb veg + 40 g hummus

Week 11 meal plan shopping list

QUANTITY	ITEM	QUANTITY	ITEM
	FRUIT		baby spinach leaves
	dried dates		baby spinach and rocket leaf mix
	lemons		tomatoes
	passionfruit		roma tomatoes
	strawberries		zucchini
	VEGETABLES		**PROTEIN**
	asparagus		lean chicken breast fillets
	avocado		lean chicken breast stir-fry strips
	bean sprouts		lean beef topside roast
	broccoli		skinless, boneless salmon fillets
	broccolini		Gruyere cheese
	cauliflower		
	celery		**OTHER**
	Chinese cabbage (wombok)		basil
	corn		chives
	Lebanese cucumbers		flat-leaf parsley
	baby fennel		mint
	baby green beans		oregano
	baby cos lettuce		rosemary
	cup mushrooms		
	red onion		pitted small Kalamata olives
	spring onions		ciabatta
	parsnips		
	potatoes		
	baby potatoes		
	pumpkin		
	baby radishes		
	baby rocket leaves		
	mixed salad leaves		

Week 12

	MONDAY	TUESDAY	WEDNESDAY	THURSDAY	FRIDAY	SATURDAY	SUNDAY
Breakfast	2 x rye Cruskits, + 20 g nut butter with no added sugar (cashew, almond or peanut) or 40 g avocado + 100 g natural Greek-style yoghurt + 30 g seeds	Scramble Pita Pockets (p 117) **UNIT TOP-UP** 100 g vanilla yoghurt (no added sugar) + 20 g raw mixed nuts	Eggplant Subs with Smashed Beans (p 161) **Carb Extra** Black coffee + 100 ml high-protein milk + 1 kiwifruit	On-the-run breakfast 1: 150 g high-protein plain yoghurt + 15 g All-Bran Original + 30 g raw mixed nuts and/or seeds **UNIT TOP-UP** Black coffee + 90 ml milk + 6 x Brazil nuts	Roasted Greens with Eggs (p 118)	Couscous Scramble (p 155)	Baked Stuffed Mushrooms (p 158)
Lunch	Cannellini Bean, Chicken and Vegetable Stew (p 179)	Cajun Tofu with Corn Salsa (p 201)	Chicken Bolognese with Konjac Spaghetti (p 193)	Salmon Salad with Seasoned Toast (p 168)	Chicken salad: Mix 50 g roast chicken + 80 g drained tinned chickpeas + 20 g grated cheddar cheese + 3 tsp olive oil + 2 tsp lime or lemon juice + 2 cups salad leaves + ½ cup sliced tomato and red onion + 30 g pumpkin seeds **Carb Extra** 1 x slice seeded low-carb bread	Mexican Fish and Black Beans (p 167) **Carb Extra** 100 g grilled sweet potato	Chicken, Cashew and Quinoa Toss (p 194)
Dinner	One-pan Lemony Chicken and Vegetables (p 217) **Carb Extra** 1 navel orange	Thai Mushroom Stir-fry with Cauliflower Omelette Rice (p 245) **Carb Extra** 1 x wholemeal mountain bread	Summer Pesto Prawns with Zucchini Noodles (p 238) **UNIT TOP-UP** 100 g vanilla yoghurt (no added sugar) + 20 g flaked almonds or raw pistachios	Smoky Pork and Barbecued Cabbage with Mustard Dressing (p 229) **Carb Extra** 100 g grilled butternut pumpkin	Vindaloo Lamb and Eggplant with Raita (p 263)	Steam-roasted Chicken with Fresh Tomato Pesto (p 221) **UNIT TOP-UP** 20 g toasted cashews	Greek Roasted Lamb Cutlets and Veggies (p 260) + 10 g raw cashews **Carb Extra** 1 small (35 g) wholegrain roll

Week 12 meal plan shopping list

QUANTITY	ITEM
	FRUIT
	kiwifruit
	lemons
	limes
	navel oranges
	VEGETABLES
	asparagus
	avocado
	baby bok choy
	broccoli
	red cabbage
	red capsicum
	carrot
	cauliflower
	Lebanese cucumbers
	eggplant
	baby green beans
	field mushrooms
	mixed mushrooms (field, portobello, shiitake, button)
	onion
	red onion
	spring onions
	butternut pumpkin
	baby radishes
	baby rocket leaves
	mixed salad leaves
	superleaf salad mix
	baby spinach leaves
	baby spinach and rocket leaf mix
	English spinach
	sweet potato
	tomatoes

QUANTITY	ITEM
	cherry tomatoes
	mixed baby tomatoes
	zucchini
	PROTEIN
	lean chicken breast fillets
	lean chicken breast stir-fry strips
	pulled roast chicken
	lean lamb backstraps
	lean pork loin steaks
	skinless, boneless flathead fillets
	cooked peeled, deveined medium tiger prawns
	OTHER
	basil
	coriander
	flat-leaf parsley
	mint
	wholegrain dinner roll

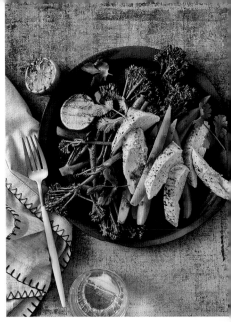

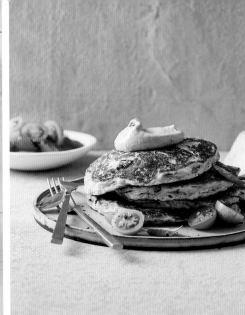

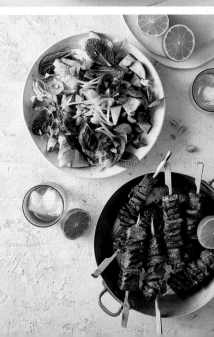

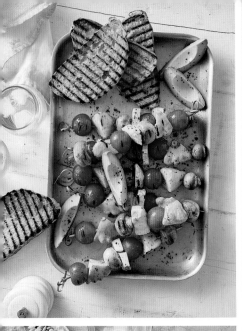

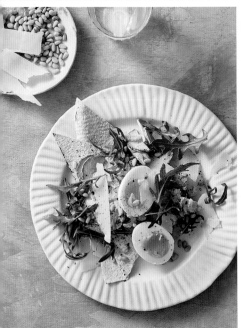

PART

4

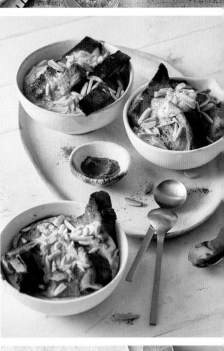

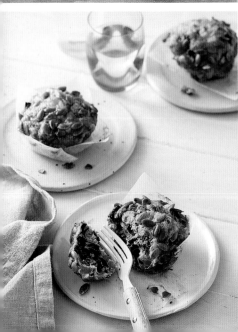

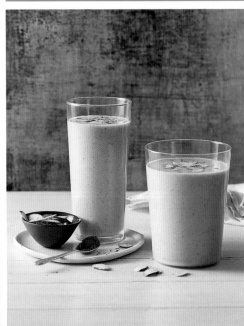

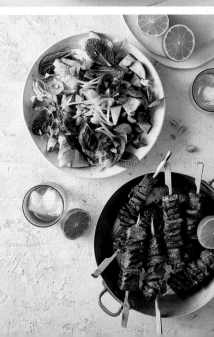

RECIPES
FOR
healthy living

1

BREAKFAST

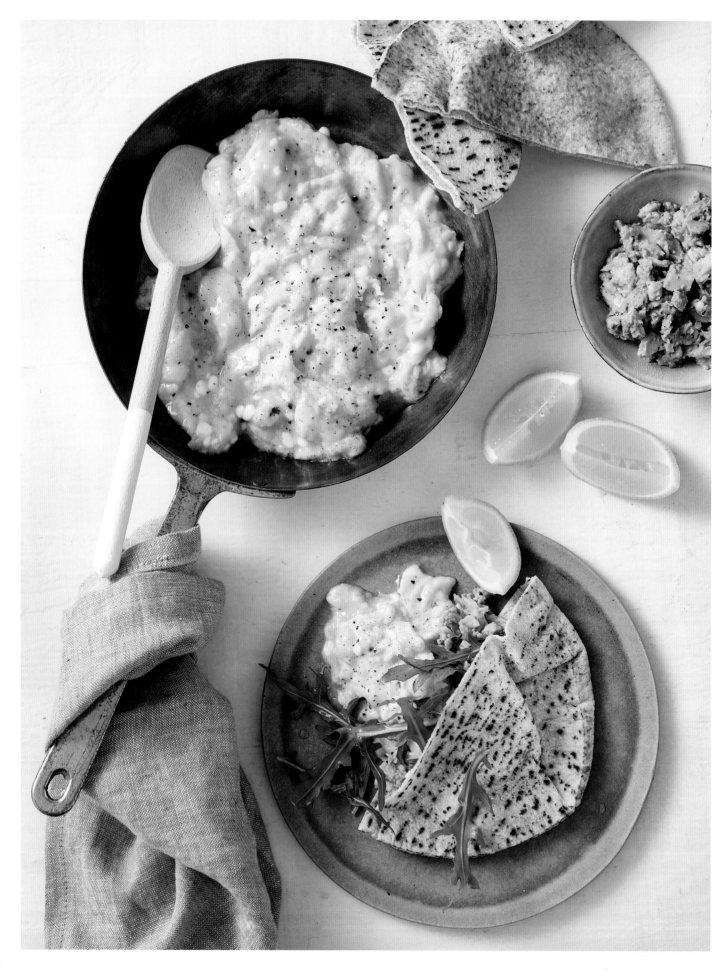

Scramble pita pockets

GRAMS CARB
9
PER SERVE

🍴 **Serves 4**   🕐 **Preparation: 15 minutes**
🍳 **Cooking: 5 minutes**   ⚙ **Difficulty: Low**

4 x 55 g eggs
1 tablespoon olive oil
80 g avocado
2 teaspoons lemon juice
2 x 35 g wholemeal pita breads,
   each halved, then split slightly
   to open pockets
220 g cottage cheese
150 g baby rocket leaves

Whisk together the eggs until well combined. Season with freshly ground black pepper.

Heat the oil in a large, non-stick frying pan over medium heat. Add the egg mixture and cook, stirring occasionally, for 2–3 minutes or until set to a firm scramble, but don't let it overcook until completely dry.

Meanwhile, mash together the avocado and lemon juice and season with freshly ground black pepper. Spread the avocado mixture evenly inside one half of each pita pocket. Fill each pita pocket with the cottage cheese and some baby rocket leaves.

Add the egg scramble mixture to the pita pockets and serve warm with the remaining rocket leaves.

UNITS PER SERVE

BREADS, CEREALS, LEGUMES, STARCHY VEGETABLES	DAIRY	LEAN MEAT, FISH, POULTRY, EGGS, TOFU	LOW-CARB VEGETABLES	MODERATE-CARB VEGETABLES	HEALTHY FATS
0.5	1	0.5	1	0	2

Roasted greens *with* eggs

🍴 Serves 4   🕐 Preparation: 20 minutes
🍲 Cooking: 20 minutes   👨‍🍳 Difficulty: Low

2 bunches asparagus, trimmed,
  diagonally halved crossways
3 zucchini, sliced into thick rounds
1 teaspoon salt-reduced garlic and
  herb seasoning
1 tablespoon olive oil
4 x 55 g eggs
⅓ cup (80 g) hummus
1 wholemeal mountain bread,
  quartered
40 g toasted unsalted pistachio
  kernels, chopped
80 g parmesan, shaved
Lemon wedges, to serve

Preheat the oven to 220°C (200°C fan-forced) and line a large baking tray with baking paper.

Add the asparagus, zucchini, seasoning and oil to the prepared tray and toss well to coat. Spread out the vegetables in a single layer and roast for 18–20 minutes or until tender and golden.

Meanwhile, cook the eggs in a saucepan of boiling water for 3–4 minutes for soft-boiled. Drain and cool slightly under cold running water, then peel and cut in half.

Divide the roasted vegetables, eggs, hummus and mountain bread among plates and sprinkle with the pistachios and parmesan. Serve with the lemon wedges.

UNITS PER SERVE					
BREADS, CEREALS, LEGUMES, STARCHY VEGETABLES	DAIRY	LEAN MEAT, FISH, POULTRY, EGGS, TOFU	LOW-CARB VEGETABLES	MODERATE-CARB VEGETABLES	HEALTHY FATS
0.5	1	0.5	1	0	2

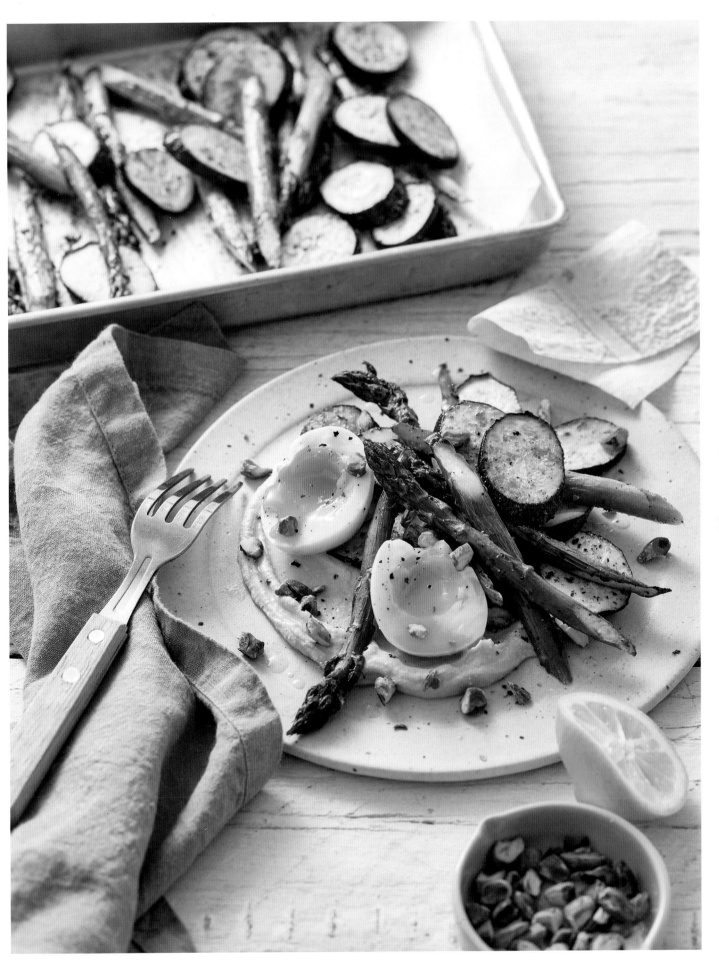

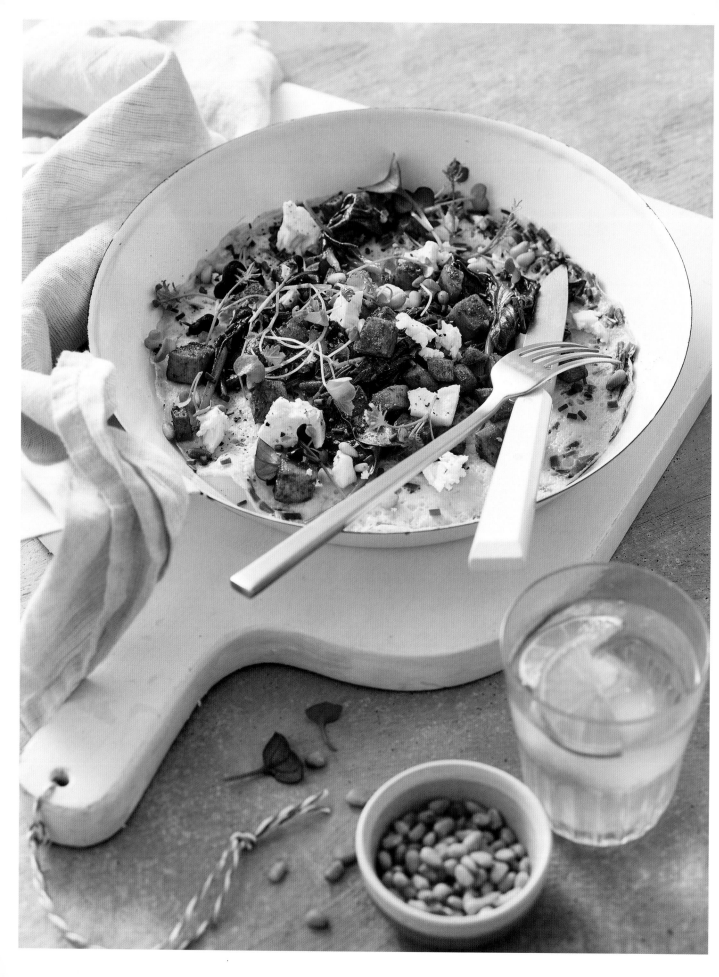

Sweet potato *and* feta omelettes

GRAMS CARB
10
PER SERVE

🍴 **Serves 4**   🕐 **Preparation: 25 minutes**
〰 **Cooking: 30 minutes**   👩‍🍳 **Difficulty: Medium**

1 tablespoon olive oil
200 g orange sweet potato,
    skin scrubbed, cubed
2 teaspoons sweet paprika
150 g baby spinach leaves
4 x 55 g eggs
2 tablespoons finely chopped chives
80 g Greek feta, crumbled
40 g toasted pine nuts
Micro herbs, to serve (optional)

Heat half the oil in a large non-stick frying pan over medium–high heat. Add the sweet potato and paprika and cook, stirring occasionally, for 8–10 minutes or until cooked and golden. Add the spinach and cook, tossing, for 30 seconds or until just wilted. Transfer the mixture to a bowl and season with freshly ground black pepper. Wipe the pan clean with paper towel.

Whisk together the eggs, chives and 1 tablespoon water in a jug and season with freshly ground black pepper.

Reheat the same pan over medium heat. Add one-quarter of the remaining oil and swirl the pan to evenly coat the base. Pour in one-quarter of the egg mixture, tilting the pan to spread it out evenly. Cook, untouched, for 3–4 minutes or until just set in the centre. Carefully slide the omelette onto a serving plate and cover to keep warm. Repeat with the remaining oil and egg mixture to make four omelettes in total.

Spoon the sweet potato mixture into the centre of the omelettes and scatter over the feta and pine nuts. Sprinkle with the micro herbs (if using) and serve.

UNITS PER SERVE					
BREADS, CEREALS, LEGUMES, STARCHY VEGETABLES	DAIRY	LEAN MEAT, FISH, POULTRY, EGGS, TOFU	LOW-CARB VEGETABLES	MODERATE-CARB VEGETABLES	HEALTHY FATS
0.5	1	0.5	<0.5	0	2

Zucchini ricotta fritters *with* basil tomatoes

GRAMS CARB
6
PER SERVE

🍴 Serves 4 🕐 Preparation: 25 minutes
🌀 Cooking: 10 minutes 👨‍🍳 Difficulty: Low

2 zucchini, coarsely grated
220 g fresh ricotta, crumbled
2 x 55 g eggs
60 g wholemeal plain flour
1 tablespoon olive oil
⅓ cup (80 g) hummus

BASIL TOMATOES
200 g mixed baby tomatoes, halved
¼ cup finely shredded basil, plus extra
   leaves to serve
1 tablespoon red wine vinegar
Pinch dried chilli flakes (optional)

To make the basil tomatoes, combine all the ingredients in a bowl. Season with freshly ground black pepper.

Mix together the zucchini, ricotta, eggs and flour in a bowl and season with freshly ground black pepper.

Heat half the oil in a large non-stick frying pan over medium–high heat. Using half the zucchini mixture, make four rounds in the hot pan. Cook for 2–3 minutes each side or until cooked and golden. Transfer the fritters to serving plates and cover to keep warm. Repeat with the remaining oil and zucchini mixture to make eight fritters in total.

Dollop hummus over the fritters, then spoon over the basil tomatoes. Garnish with the extra basil leaves and serve.

UNITS PER SERVE					
BREADS, CEREALS, LEGUMES, STARCHY VEGETABLES	DAIRY	LEAN MEAT, FISH, POULTRY, EGGS, TOFU	LOW-CARB VEGETABLES	MODERATE-CARB VEGETABLES	HEALTHY FATS
1	1	0.5	1	0	2

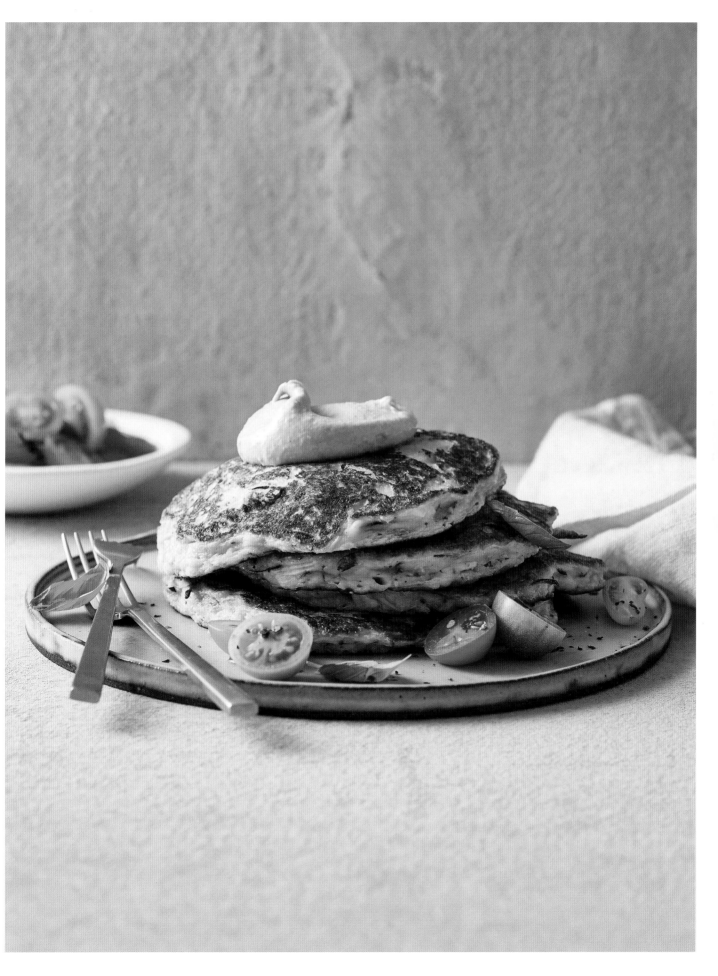

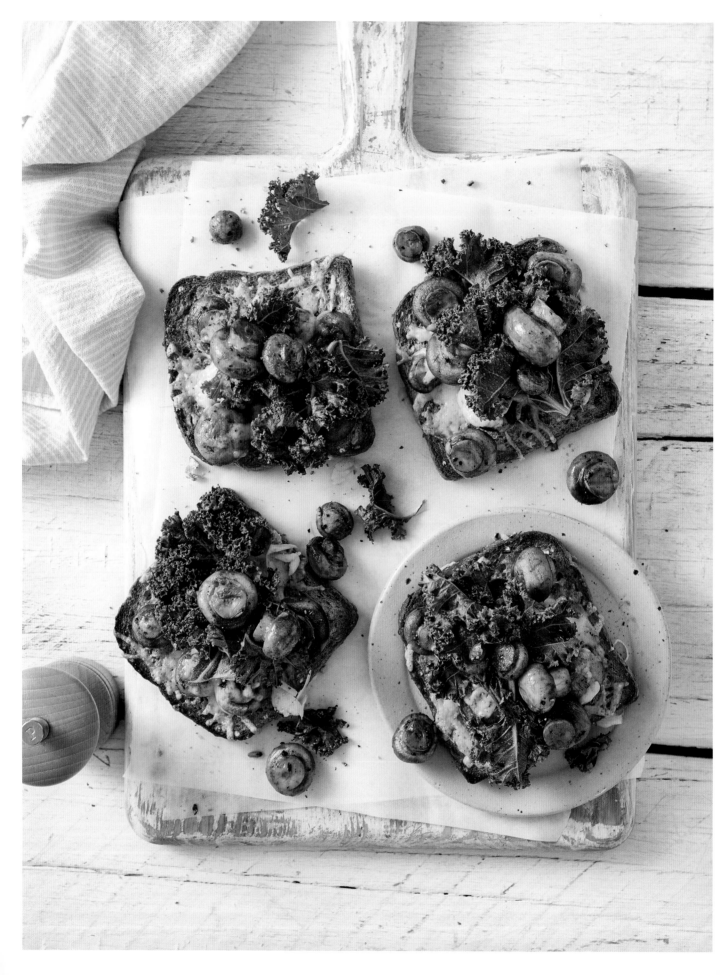

Chargrilled kale, mushroom *and* cheese open toasties

GRAMS CARB
11
PER SERVE

🍴 Serves 4   🕐 Preparation: 15 minutes
🍳 Cooking: 10 minutes   🎚 Difficulty: Low

4 kale leaves, white stalks removed
400 g button mushrooms, wiped
   clean, thickly sliced
4 x 35 g slices multigrain bread
2 tablespoons olive oil margarine
80 g Gruyere cheese, finely grated

Preheat the oven grill to high and line a baking tray with foil.

Heat a large chargrill pan over high heat. Add the kale and mushroom and cook, turning occasionally, for 3–5 minutes or until cooked and dark golden.

Place the bread slices on the prepared tray and toast on one side for 1–2 minutes or until golden. Turn them over and spread with the margarine. Top with the chargrilled kale and mushroom and then the cheese.

Cook under the grill for 1–2 minutes or until the cheese is melted and golden. Serve immediately.

UNITS PER SERVE

BREADS, CEREALS, LEGUMES, STARCHY VEGETABLES	DAIRY	LEAN MEAT, FISH, POULTRY, EGGS, TOFU	LOW-CARB VEGETABLES	MODERATE-CARB VEGETABLES	HEALTHY FATS
1	1	0	1	0	2

Herb-stuffed eggs

GRAMS CARB
16
PER SERVE

🍴 Serves 4　🕐 Preparation: 20 minutes
🍲 Cooking: 10 minutes　🥄 Difficulty: Low

MAKE AHEAD　**PORTABLE**

4 x 55 g eggs
⅓ cup (80 g) hummus
80 g parmesan, grated
80 g avocado
1 tablespoon lemon juice
1 tablespoon finely chopped chives
150 g baby rocket leaves
8 multigrain Ryvitas, broken in half

Cook the eggs in a saucepan of boiling water for 6–7 minutes for hard-boiled. Drain and cool slightly under cold running water, then peel and cut in half lengthways.

Scoop out the egg yolks and place in a bowl. Add the hummus, parmesan, avocado, lemon juice and chives, season with freshly ground black pepper and mash until smooth. Spoon the mixture into the egg white cavities.

Divide the stuffed eggs, rocket and Ryvitas among plates and serve.

Notes:
▶ If making ahead, store the stuffed eggs in an airtight container in the fridge for up to 3 days.

▶ To make it portable, store the stuffed eggs, Ryvitas and rocket leaves in separate airtight containers. Keep cool while transporting.

UNITS PER SERVE

BREADS, CEREALS, LEGUMES, STARCHY VEGETABLES	DAIRY	LEAN MEAT, FISH, POULTRY, EGGS, TOFU	LOW-CARB VEGETABLES	MODERATE-CARB VEGETABLES	HEALTHY FATS
0.5	1	0.5	0.5	0	2

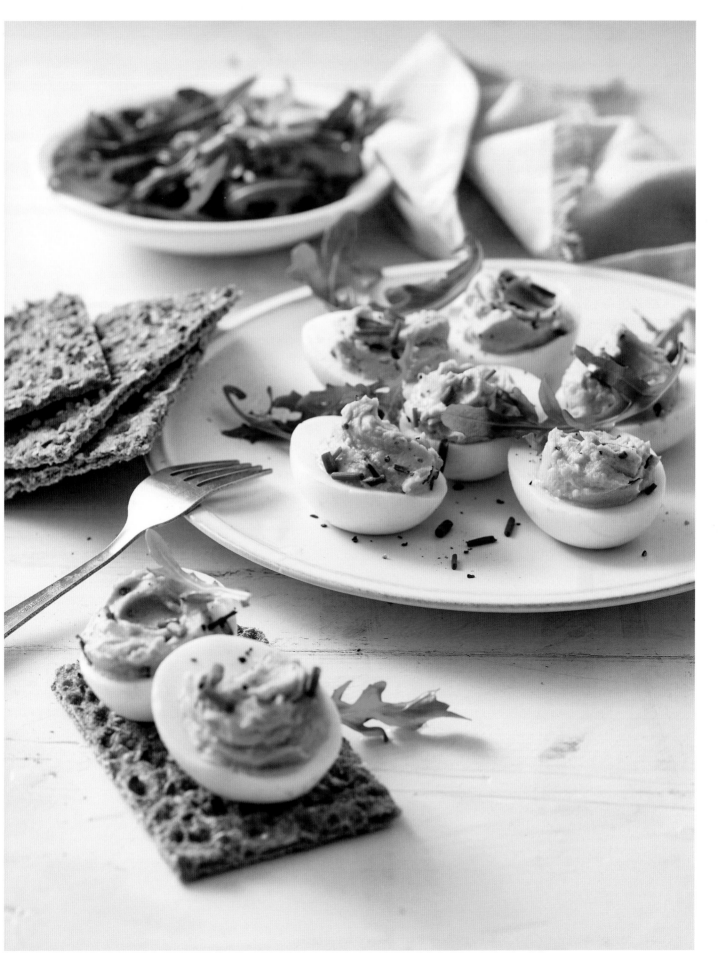

Bruschetta *with* bocconcini *and* pecans

(21) GRAMS CARB PER SERVE

🍴 Serves 4   🕐 Preparation: 10 minutes, plus 15 minutes standing time
👨‍🍳 Difficulty: Low

1 tablespoon extra virgin olive oil
1 tablespoon balsamic vinegar
4 tomatoes, sliced into rounds
½ cup basil leaves, torn, plus extra small leaves to serve
4 x 35 g slices ciabatta, toasted
100 g baby bocconcini, torn
40 g toasted pecans, chopped

Whisk together the oil and vinegar in a bowl and season with freshly ground black pepper. Add the tomato and torn basil leaves. Stand at room temperature, tossing occasionally, for 15 minutes to macerate.

Divide the hot toast among plates. Top with the tomato mixture, then the bocconcini. Sprinkle with the pecans and extra basil leaves and serve.

UNITS PER SERVE

BREADS, CEREALS, LEGUMES, STARCHY VEGETABLES	DAIRY	LEAN MEAT, FISH, POULTRY, EGGS, TOFU	LOW-CARB VEGETABLES	MODERATE-CARB VEGETABLES	HEALTHY FATS
1	1	0	1	0	2

Loaded breakfast beans

GRAMS CARB
22
PER SERVE

🍴 Serves 4   🕐 Preparation: 15 minutes
🍳 Cooking: 10 minutes, plus 5 minutes standing time   Difficulty: Low

MAKE AHEAD   **PORTABLE**

1 tablespoon olive oil
2 cloves garlic, crushed
2 zucchini, chopped
2 spring onions, sliced
2 overripe tomatoes, chopped
300 g jar mild chunky tomato salsa
400 g drained, rinsed tinned
    cannellini beans (see note)
2 bunches asparagus, trimmed
80 g avocado, sliced
80 g sharp cheddar, crumbled
Lime wedges, to serve (optional)

Heat the oil in a large deep non-stick frying pan over medium–high heat. Add the garlic, zucchini and spring onion and cook, stirring occasionally, for 5 minutes or until softened and golden.

Add the tomato, salsa and cannellini beans and cook, stirring occasionally, for 5 minutes or until the sauce has reduced by half. Remove the pan from the heat and add the asparagus, then stand, covered, for 5 minutes.

Top the loaded beans with the avocado and cheddar and serve straight from the pan with the lime wedges alongside (if using).

Notes: You will require 2 x 400 g tins of cannellini beans for this recipe. Store leftover beans in an airtight container in the fridge for up to 3 days.

❱ If making ahead, store the slightly cooled bean mixture in an airtight container in the fridge for up to 3 days. Reheat gently over low heat, adding a little water to loosen the mixture if necessary.

❱ To make it portable, store the beans, avocado and lime wedges in separate airtight containers. Keep cool while transporting. The beans are delicious heated or at room temperature.

UNITS PER SERVE

BREADS, CEREALS, LEGUMES, STARCHY VEGETABLES	DAIRY	LEAN MEAT, FISH, POULTRY, EGGS, TOFU	LOW-CARB VEGETABLES	MODERATE-CARB VEGETABLES	HEALTHY FATS
1	1	0	1	1	2

Spinach *and* cheddar bakes

GRAMS CARB
12
PER SERVE

🍴 Serves 4 (makes 8)   🕐 Preparation: 20 minutes
♨ Cooking: 25 minutes, plus 10 minutes resting time   ⊙ Difficulty: Low

(MAKE AHEAD)   (PORTABLE)

150 g baby spinach leaves
Boiling water, for blanching
4 x 55 g eggs, whisked
1 tablespoon basil pesto
2 tomatoes, finely chopped
60 g wholemeal self-raising flour
80 g mild cheddar, grated
40 g pumpkin seeds (pepitas)

Preheat the oven to 200°C (180°C fan-forced). Line eight holes of a 12-hole, ⅓ cup muffin tin with paper cases.

Place the spinach in a colander in the sink and pour over boiling water until it has wilted. Cool and refresh under cold running water. Squeeze out the excess water and pat dry with paper towel, then finely chop.

Place the spinach, egg, pesto, tomato, flour and half the cheddar in a bowl and stir until just combined. Season with freshly ground black pepper. Divide the mixture evenly among the prepared muffin holes and sprinkle the pumpkin seeds and remaining cheddar over the top.

Bake for 20–25 minutes or until cooked, puffed and golden. Rest in the tin for 10 minutes, then carefully remove. Serve warm or at room temperature.

Notes:
▶ If making ahead, store the cooled bakes in an airtight container in the fridge for up to 3 days. Serve cold or warm through in the oven at 150°C (130°C fan-forced).

▶ Make it portable by storing the bakes in an airtight container. Keep cool while transporting.

UNITS PER SERVE					
BREADS, CEREALS, LEGUMES, STARCHY VEGETABLES	DAIRY	LEAN MEAT, FISH, POULTRY, EGGS, TOFU	LOW-CARB VEGETABLES	MODERATE-CARB VEGETABLES	HEALTHY FATS
1	1	0.5	1	0	2

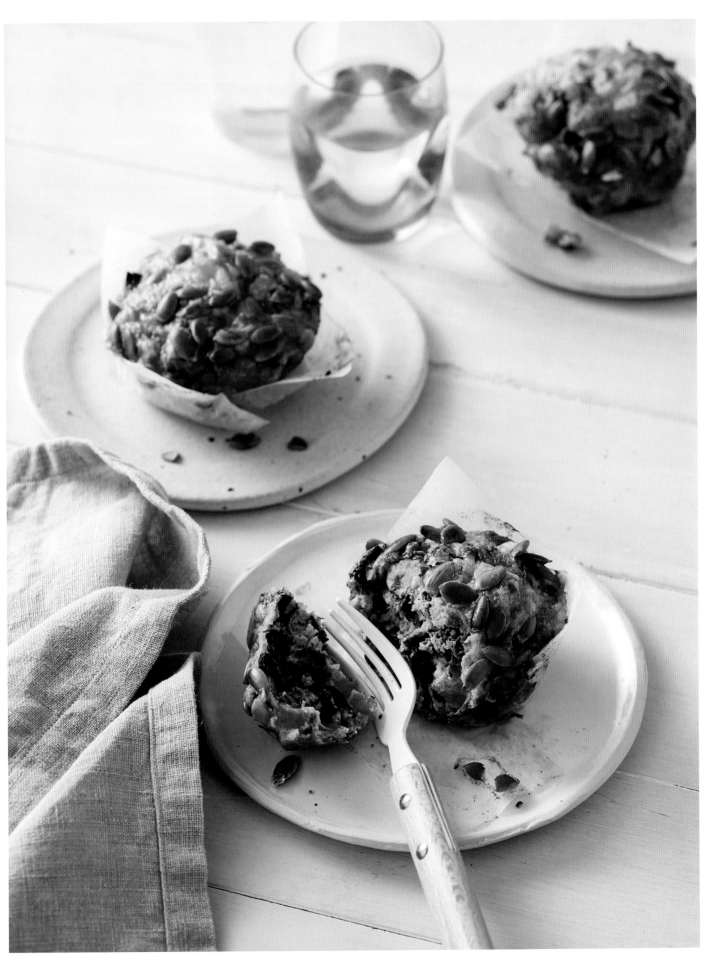

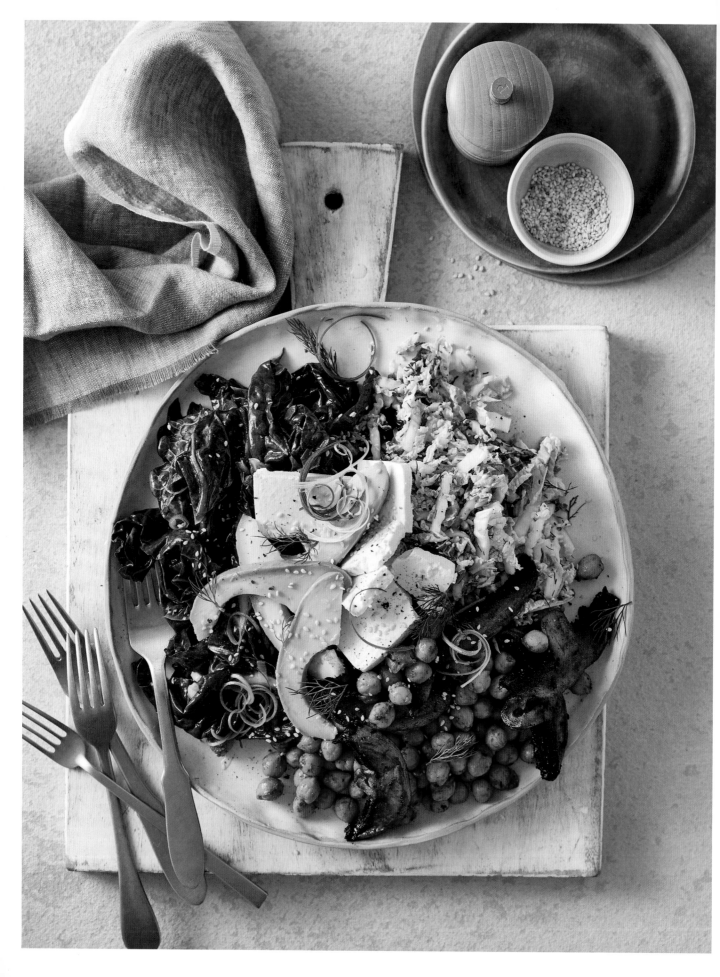

Breakfast plate

GRAMS CARB
12
PER SERVE

🍽 **Serves 4**   ⏱ **Preparation: 30 minutes, plus 1 hour standing time**
♨ **Cooking: 15 minutes**   🍲 **Difficulty: Low**

WEEKEND FOOD

1 tablespoon olive oil

1 clove garlic, crushed

320 g drained, rinsed tinned
    chickpeas (see note)

2 teaspoons smoked paprika

4 large field mushrooms, wiped clean,
    thickly sliced

2 spring onions, sliced

1 bunch silverbeet, white stalks
    removed and leaves torn

60 g avocado, sliced

80 g Danish feta, crumbled

1 tablespoon toasted sesame seeds

PICKLED CABBAGE

¼ cup (60 ml) red wine vinegar

2 teaspoons wholegrain mustard

1 tablespoon dill fronds, plus extra
    to serve

200 g wombok (Chinese cabbage),
    very thinly sliced

To make the pickled cabbage, combine all the ingredients in a bowl. Cover and stand at room temperature for 1 hour, stirring occasionally.

Heat half the oil in a large non-stick frying pan over medium heat. Add the garlic, chickpeas and paprika and cook, tossing occasionally, for 10 minutes or until golden and heated through. Transfer to a bowl. Return the pan to the heat, add the mushroom and cook, tossing, for 5 minutes or until just softened and golden.

Meanwhile, heat the remaining oil in a large deep saucepan over high heat, add two-thirds of the spring onion and all the silverbeet and cook, covered and stirring occasionally, for 5–6 minutes or until wilted. Season with freshly ground black pepper.

Divide the chickpeas, mushroom, silverbeet mixture and pickled cabbage among plates. Sprinkle with the avocado, feta, remaining spring onion, dill and sesame seeds.

Notes: You will require 2 x 400 g tins of chickpeas for this recipe. Store leftover chickpeas in an airtight container in the fridge for up to 3 days.

▶ If making the pickled cabbage ahead, store the mixture in an airtight container in the fridge for up to 3 days, stirring occasionally. The cabbage will soften and lose a little of its green vibrancy over time, so add more fresh dill if desired.

UNITS PER SERVE

BREADS, CEREALS, LEGUMES, STARCHY VEGETABLES	DAIRY	LEAN MEAT, FISH, POULTRY, EGGS, TOFU	LOW-CARB VEGETABLES	MODERATE-CARB VEGETABLES	HEALTHY FATS
1	1	0	2	1	2

Individual fruit toast puddings

GRAMS CARB
19
PER SERVE

🍴 Serves 4   🕐 Preparation: 25 minutes, plus 10 minutes standing time
♨ Cooking: 20 minutes   🌡 Difficulty: Low

WEEKEND FOOD

1 tablespoon olive oil margarine
4 x 30 g slices fruit bread
4 x 55 g eggs
200 g Greek-style yoghurt
1 teaspoon artificial sweetener
   (stevia powder)
1 teaspoon ground cinnamon
110 g fresh ricotta, crumbled
40 g slivered almonds

Preheat the oven to 180°C (160°C fan-forced). Using 1 teaspoon of the margarine, lightly grease four ¾ cup ramekins. Spread the remaining margarine evenly over one side of each slice of bread, then cut each slice into four triangles.

Whisk the eggs, yoghurt, sweetener, cinnamon and half the ricotta in a bowl until well combined.

Divide the bread pieces among the prepared ramekins, then evenly pour over the egg mixture. Sprinkle with the remaining ricotta, then the almonds.

Bake for 15–18 minutes or until the egg is firmly set and the tops are golden. Serve.

UNITS PER SERVE

BREADS, CEREALS, LEGUMES, STARCHY VEGETABLES	DAIRY	LEAN MEAT, FISH, POULTRY, EGGS, TOFU	LOW-CARB VEGETABLES	MODERATE-CARB VEGETABLES	HEALTHY FATS
1	1	0.5	0	0	2

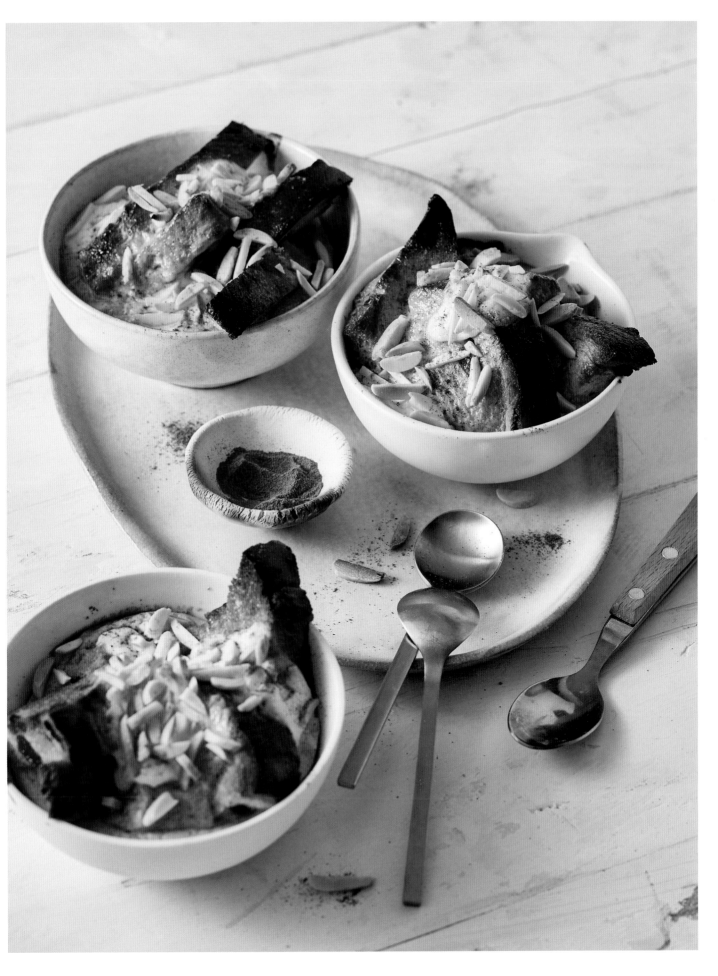

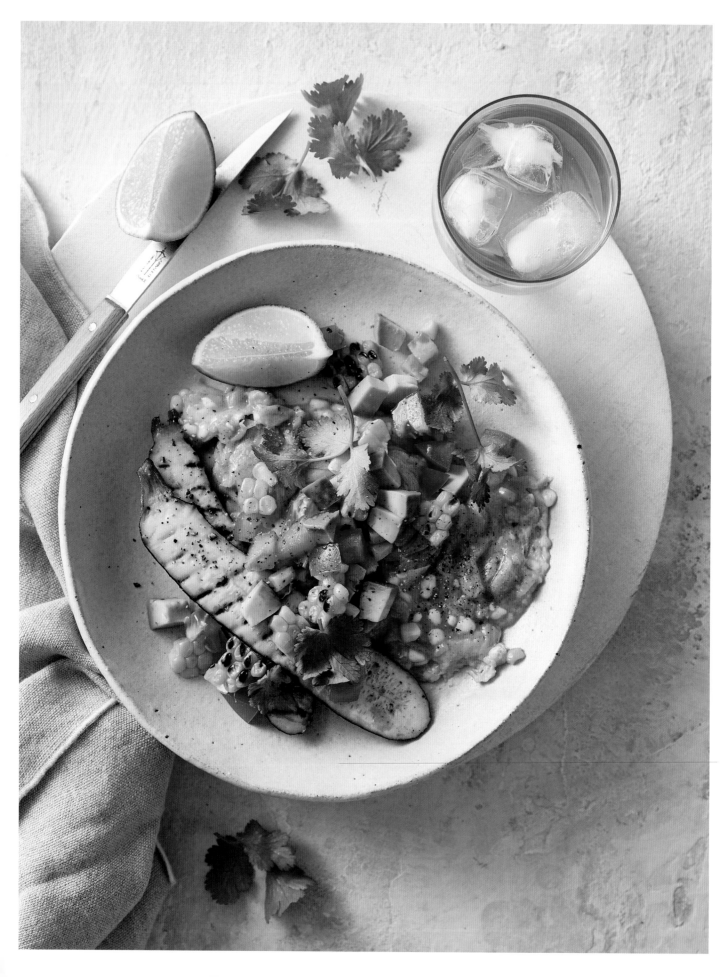

Tex-mex scramble
with chargrilled corn salsa

GRAMS CARB
14
PER SERVE

🍴 Serves 4   🕐 Preparation: 25 minutes
♨ Cooking: 20 minutes   👨‍🍳 Difficulty: Low

WEEKEND FOOD

4 zucchini, each cut lengthways
    into thirds
4 x 55 g eggs
110 g cottage cheese
40 g Danish feta, crumbled
2 teaspoons Mexican seasoning
1 tablespoon olive oil

CHARGRILLED CORN SALSA
1 corn cob, husk and silks removed
2 tomatoes, chopped
80 g avocado, chopped
¼ cup coriander sprigs, torn
Finely grated zest and juice of 1 lime,
    plus lime wedges to serve

To make the chargrilled corn salsa, preheat a chargrill pan over high heat. Add the corn and cook, turning occasionally, for 6–8 minutes or until just cooked and golden. Transfer to a board, then carefully slice off the kernels. Transfer the kernels to a bowl and add all the remaining ingredients. Season with freshly ground black pepper and stir to combine, then set aside until ready to serve.

Reheat the chargrill pan over high heat. Add the zucchini and cook, turning occasionally, for 8–10 minutes or until cooked and deep golden.

Meanwhile, whisk the eggs, cottage cheese, feta and Mexican seasoning in a bowl.

Heat the oil in a large non-stick frying pan over high heat. Add the egg mixture and cook, stirring gently occasionally, for 1–2 minutes or until softly set.

Spoon the scramble onto plates and arrange the zucchini alongside. Add the corn salsa and serve with the lime wedges.

UNITS PER SERVE

BREADS, CEREALS, LEGUMES, STARCHY VEGETABLES	DAIRY	LEAN MEAT, FISH, POULTRY, EGGS, TOFU	LOW-CARB VEGETABLES	MODERATE-CARB VEGETABLES	HEALTHY FATS
0.5	1	0.5	2	0	2

Frozen cereal *and* yoghurt discs

GRAMS CARB
21
PER SERVE

🍴 Serves 4 (makes 12)   🕐 Preparation: 15 minutes, plus 2 hours freezing time
🍲 Difficulty: Low

MAKE AHEAD

400 g Greek-style yoghurt
1 teaspoon ground ginger
120 g Freedom Foods cranberry,
    almond and cinnamon cereal
80 g toasted pumpkin seeds (pepitas)

Line two large baking trays with baking paper.

Whisk the yoghurt and ginger in a bowl until well combined. Dollop the mixture onto the prepared trays to form twelve 7 cm rounds. Sprinkle the tops with the cereal and pumpkin seeds.

Freeze for 2 hours or until firm. Serve straight away or transfer the discs to an airtight container, layered between pieces of baking paper, and store in the freezer for up to 3 months.

UNITS PER SERVE

BREADS, CEREALS, LEGUMES, STARCHY VEGETABLES	DAIRY	LEAN MEAT, FISH, POULTRY, EGGS, TOFU	LOW-CARB VEGETABLES	MODERATE-CARB VEGETABLES	HEALTHY FATS
1	1	0	0	0	2

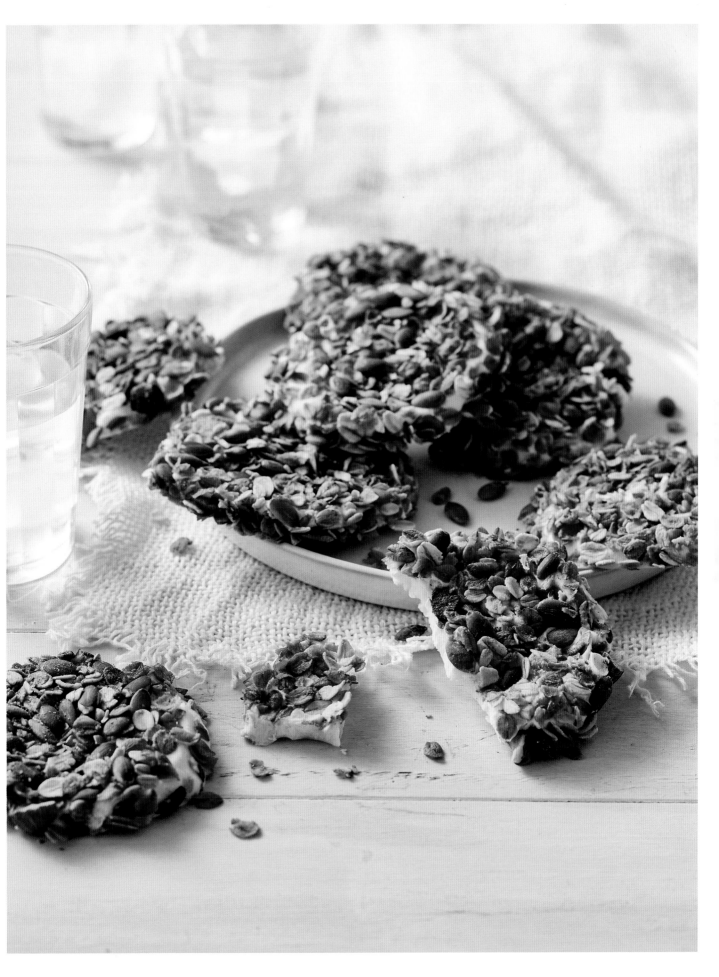

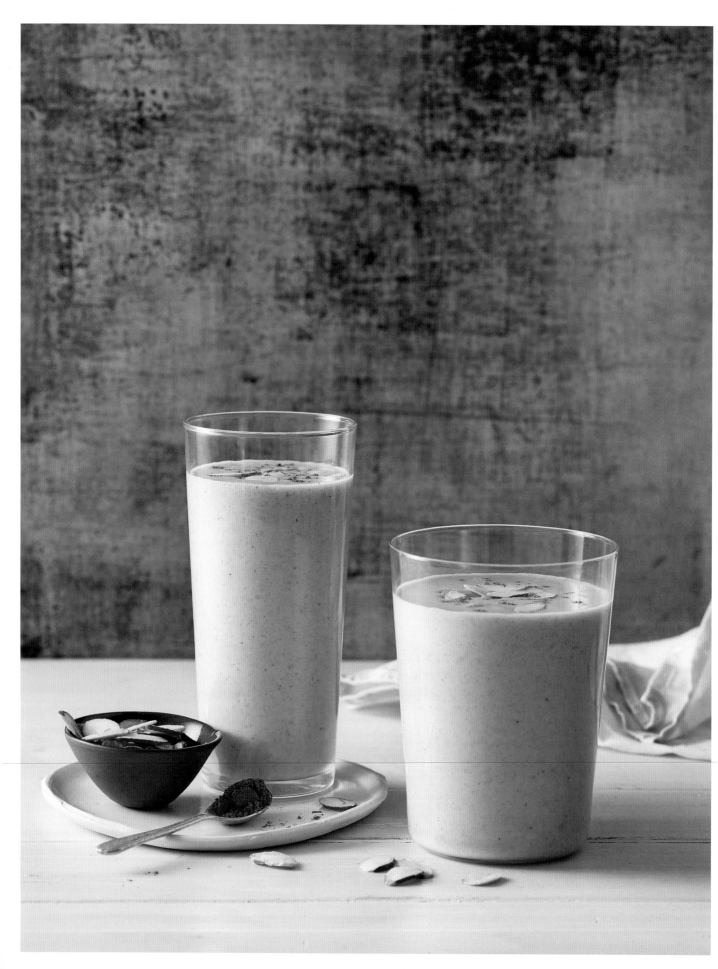

Oat *and* almond caramel shake

GRAMS CARB **23** *PER SERVE*

🍴 Serves 4   🕐 Preparation: 10 minutes, plus 5 minutes cooling time
〰 Cooking: 15 minutes   💡 Difficulty: Low

120 g rolled oats
2 teaspoons mixed spice, plus extra
   for sprinkling
1 tablespoon diet caramel topping
600 ml calcium-enriched almond milk
200 g Greek-style yoghurt
80 g toasted flaked almonds

Place the oats, mixed spice and 2 cups (500 ml) water in a small saucepan over medium–low heat. Cook, stirring occasionally, for 12–15 minutes or until softened and the water has reduced by half. Cool in the pan for 5 minutes, then transfer to an upright blender.

Add the caramel topping, almond milk and yoghurt to the blender and blitz on high speed until completely smooth. Pour into tall serving glasses, sprinkle with the flaked almonds and a little extra mixed spice, and serve.

UNITS PER SERVE

BREADS, CEREALS, LEGUMES, STARCHY VEGETABLES	DAIRY	LEAN MEAT, FISH, POULTRY, EGGS, TOFU	LOW-CARB VEGETABLES	MODERATE-CARB VEGETABLES	HEALTHY FATS
1	1	0	0	0	2

Quinoa breakfast bowls

GRAMS CARB
16
PER SERVE

🍴 Serves 4   🕐 Preparation: 25 minutes
♨ Cooking: 25 minutes   🖐 Difficulty: Medium

WEEKEND FOOD

80 g quinoa, rinsed well and drained
1 tablespoon olive oil
1 long green chilli, seeded and
   thinly sliced
1 bunch kale, white stalks removed,
   leaves thickly sliced
80 g haloumi, sliced
4 x 55 g eggs
80 g avocado, sliced
Micro herbs and lemon wedges,
   to serve (optional)

TAHINI DRIZZLE
1 tablespoon hulled tahini
Finely grated zest and juice of
   1 large lemon
2 teaspoons warm water
1 teaspoon sweet paprika

To make the tahini drizzle, whisk together all the ingredients in a small bowl. Season with freshly ground black pepper. Set aside at room temperature until you are ready to serve. (This will thicken on standing so you may need to add a little more warm water just before serving.)

Cook the quinoa in a saucepan of boiling water for 12–15 minutes or until tender. Drain and refresh under cold running water, then transfer to a large bowl and set aside.

Heat the oil in a large deep non-stick frying pan over high heat. Add the chilli and kale and cook, tossing, for 4–5 minutes or until wilted and starting to crisp. Tip into the bowl with the quinoa, then reheat the pan over high heat. Add the haloumi and cook, turning occasionally for 1–2 minutes or until golden. Transfer to the bowl with the quinoa. Season with freshly ground black pepper, then cover loosely to keep warm.

Meanwhile, poach the eggs (in two batches) in a large saucepan of gently simmering water for 1–2 minutes or until the egg whites are just set but the yolks are still runny. Carefully remove with a slotted spoon and drain on paper towel.

Divide the quinoa, kale and haloumi mixture among serving bowls. Place a poached egg on top, then spoon over the tahini drizzle. Finish with the avocado and micro herbs (if using) and serve with the lemon wedges.

UNITS PER SERVE

BREADS, CEREALS, LEGUMES, STARCHY VEGETABLES	DAIRY	LEAN MEAT, FISH, POULTRY, EGGS, TOFU	LOW-CARB VEGETABLES	MODERATE-CARB VEGETABLES	HEALTHY FATS
1	1	0.5	1	0	2

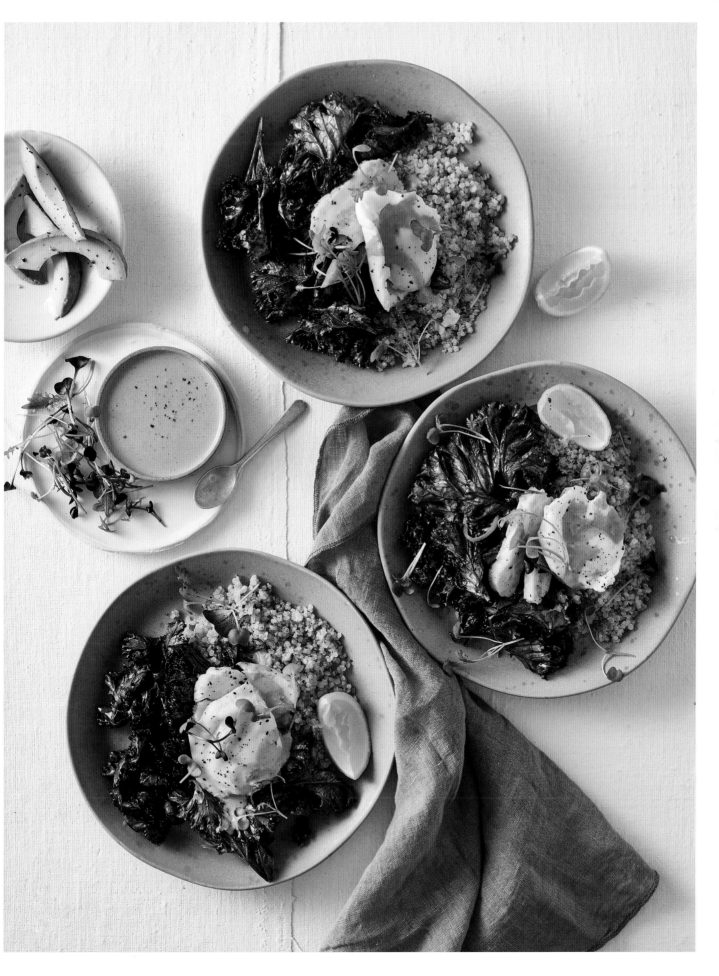

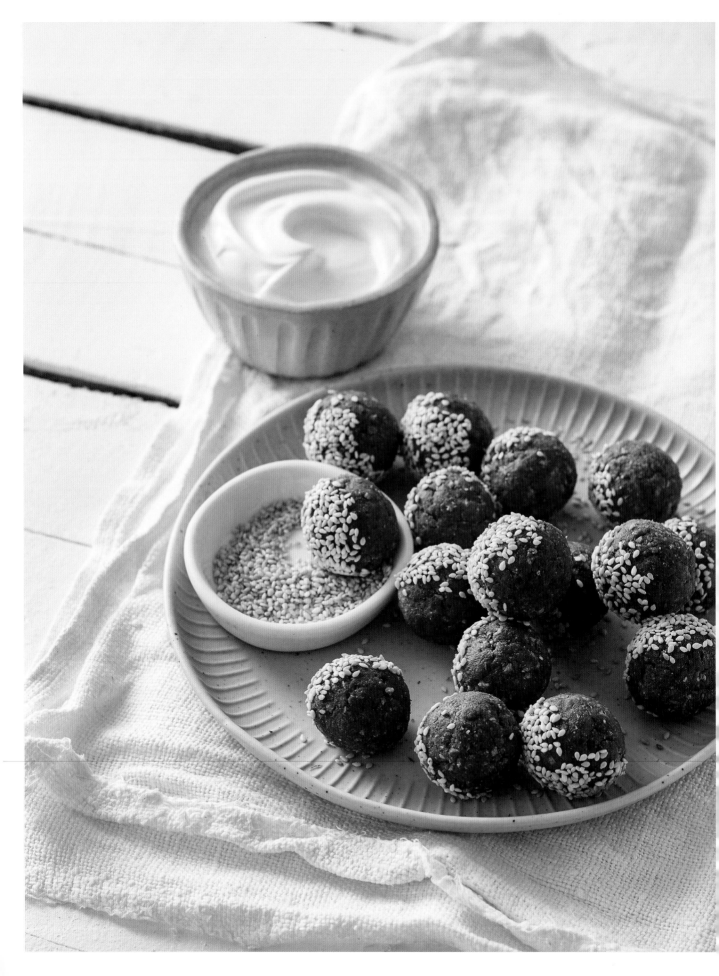

Weet-Bix *and* yoghurt bliss balls

GRAMS CARB
(23)
PER SERVE

🍴 **Serves 4 (makes 20)**   🕐 **Preparation: 20 minutes, plus 20 minutes chilling time**
👨‍🍳 **Difficulty: Low**

MAKE AHEAD

120 g Hi-Bran Weet-Bix, broken
1 tablespoon cocoa powder
2 teaspoons artificial sweetener
    (stevia powder) (optional)
1 tablespoon almond butter (see note)
200 g Greek-style yoghurt, plus extra
    200 g to serve
40 g toasted sesame seeds

Blitz the Weet-Bix, cocoa and sweetener (if using) in a food processor until finely chopped. Add the almond butter and yoghurt and blend until well combined. Transfer the mixture to the fridge for 20 minutes or until chilled and firm.

Roll 1 tablespoon measures of the mixture into balls, then lightly dip the tops into the sesame seeds. Serve with the extra yoghurt for dipping.

Notes: It is important to use a good-quality thick almond butter for this recipe – even better if your local health-food shop grinds fresh nuts into a butter.

▶ If making ahead, store the balls in an airtight container in the fridge for up to 5 days. Serve chilled.

UNITS PER SERVE

BREADS, CEREALS, LEGUMES, STARCHY VEGETABLES	DAIRY	LEAN MEAT, FISH, POULTRY, EGGS, TOFU	LOW-CARB VEGETABLES	MODERATE-CARB VEGETABLES	HEALTHY FATS
1	1	0	1	0	2

Lentil breakfast bowls

GRAMS CARB
15
PER SERVE

🍴 Serves 4   🕐 Preparation: 20 minutes
🌀 Cooking: 15 minutes   👨‍🍳 Difficulty: Medium

WEEKEND FOOD

360 g drained, rinsed tinned
   lentils (see note)
½ cup small mint leaves
¼ cup chopped flat-leaf parsley
1 bunch watercress, trimmed
4 roma tomatoes, quartered
   lengthways
80 g goat's feta, crumbled
Lemon wedges, to serve

DRESSING
1 teaspoon sumac (see note)
2 tablespoons extra virgin olive oil
Finely grated zest and juice of 1 lemon

Preheat the oven to 200°C (180°C fan-forced).

To make the dressing, whisk together all the ingredients in a large
bowl. Season with freshly ground black pepper.

Combine the lentils and dressing in a bowl and toss well to combine.
Set aside, tossing occasionally, until you are ready to serve.

Add the mint, parsley, watercress and tomato to the lentil mixture
and gently toss to combine. Divide among bowls and sprinkle with
the feta.

Notes: You will require 2 x 400 g tins of lentils for this recipe.
Store any leftover lentils in an airtight container in the fridge for
up to 3 days.

▶ Sumac is a mild spice with a lemony flavour. It is readily available
in supermarkets, but you can use sweet paprika instead, if preferred.

UNITS PER SERVE

BREADS, CEREALS, LEGUMES, STARCHY VEGETABLES	DAIRY	LEAN MEAT, FISH, POULTRY, EGGS, TOFU	LOW-CARB VEGETABLES	MODERATE-CARB VEGETABLES	HEALTHY FATS
1	1	0	1	0	2

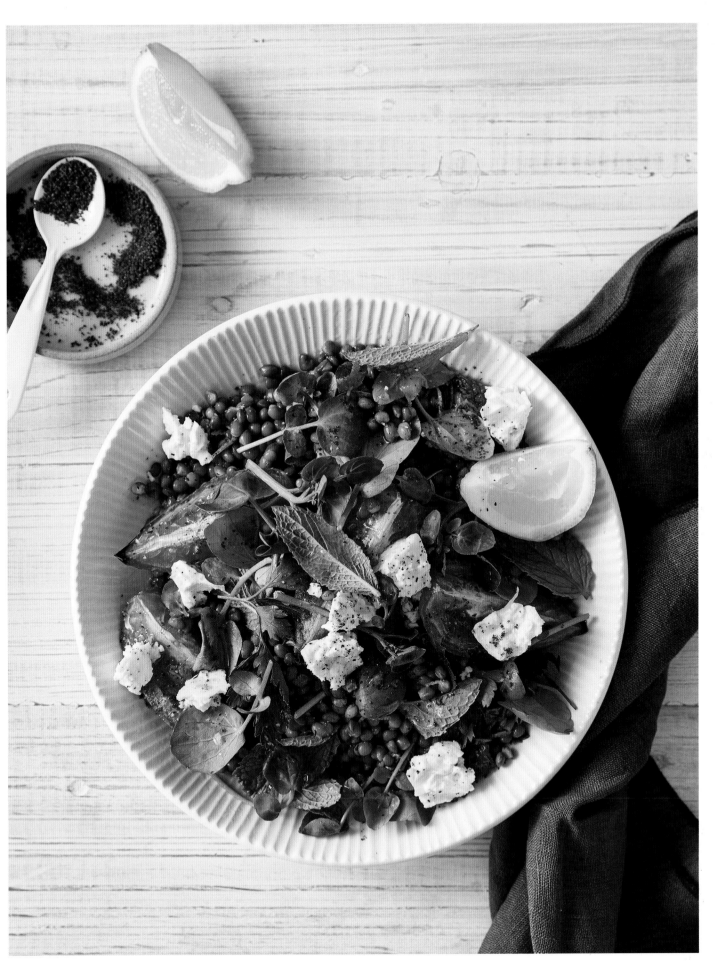

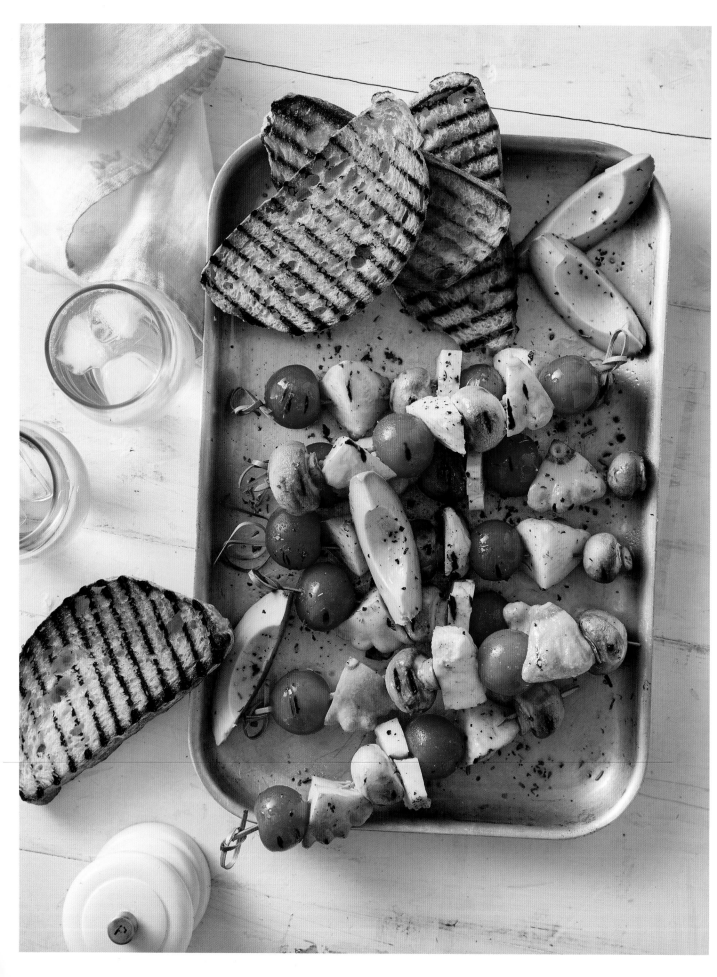

Marinated breakfast kebabs

GRAMS CARB
18
PER SERVE

🍴 Serves 4   🕐 35 minutes, plus 1 hour marinating time
♨ Cooking: 15 minutes   👨‍🍳 Difficulty: Medium

WEEKEND FOOD   MAKE AHEAD

4 baby yellow squash, quartered
16 button mushrooms
250 g cherry tomatoes
80 g haloumi, cut into 8 pieces
80 g avocado, sliced
4 x 35 g slices ciabatta, toasted

MARINADE
1 tablespoon extra virgin olive oil
1 tablespoon red wine vinegar
1 teaspoon dried mixed herbs
1 small clove garlic, crushed

Soak eight bamboo skewers in water for 20 minutes.

To make the marinade, whisk together all the ingredients in a large flat glass or ceramic dish. Season with freshly ground black pepper.

Thread the squash, mushrooms, tomatoes and haloumi alternately onto the skewers. Place skewers in the marinade dish and turn to coat on all sides. Cover and chill, turning occasionally, for 1 hour or overnight if time permits.

Preheat a barbecue chargrill plate to medium–high. Cook the skewers, turning occasionally, for 8–10 minutes or until just cooked and golden.

Divide the avocado and toasted ciabatta among plates. Add the vegetable kebabs and serve.

UNITS PER SERVE

BREADS, CEREALS, LEGUMES, STARCHY VEGETABLES	DAIRY	LEAN MEAT, FISH, POULTRY, EGGS, TOFU	LOW-CARB VEGETABLES	MODERATE-CARB VEGETABLES	HEALTHY FATS
1	1	0	2	0	2

Poached eggs *with* veggies *and* pesto parmesan yoghurt

GRAMS CARB
11
PER SERVE

🍴 Serves 4   🕐 Preparation: 20 minutes
⊛ Cooking: 15 minutes   ⊜ Difficulty: Medium

WEEKEND FOOD

3 zucchini, quartered lengthways

3 bunches asparagus, trimmed

4 x 55 g eggs

40 g toasted pumpkin seeds (pepitas)

2 x 35 g multigrain bread slices,
   toasted and halved

PESTO PARMESAN YOGHURT

60 g parmesan, very finely grated

100 g Greek-style yoghurt

Finely grated zest and juice of
   1 small lemon

1 tablespoon basil pesto

To make the pesto parmesan yoghurt, combine all the ingredients in a bowl. Season with freshly ground black pepper, then cover and chill until required.

Preheat a large chargrill pan over high heat. Add the zucchini and asparagus in two batches and cook, turning occasionally, for 5–7 minutes each or until just tender and golden. Arrange on a serving platter and spoon the pesto parmesan yoghurt alongside.

Meanwhile, poach the eggs (in two batches) in a large saucepan of gently simmering water for 1–2 minutes or until the egg whites are just set but the yolks are still runny. Carefully remove with a slotted spoon and drain on paper towel.

Place the poached eggs on top of the vegetables and pesto parmesan yoghurt, sprinkle with the pumpkin seeds and serve with the toast.

UNITS PER SERVE

BREADS, CEREALS, LEGUMES, STARCHY VEGETABLES	DAIRY	LEAN MEAT, FISH, POULTRY, EGGS, TOFU	LOW-CARB VEGETABLES	MODERATE-CARB VEGETABLES	HEALTHY FATS
0.5	1	0.5	1.5	0	2

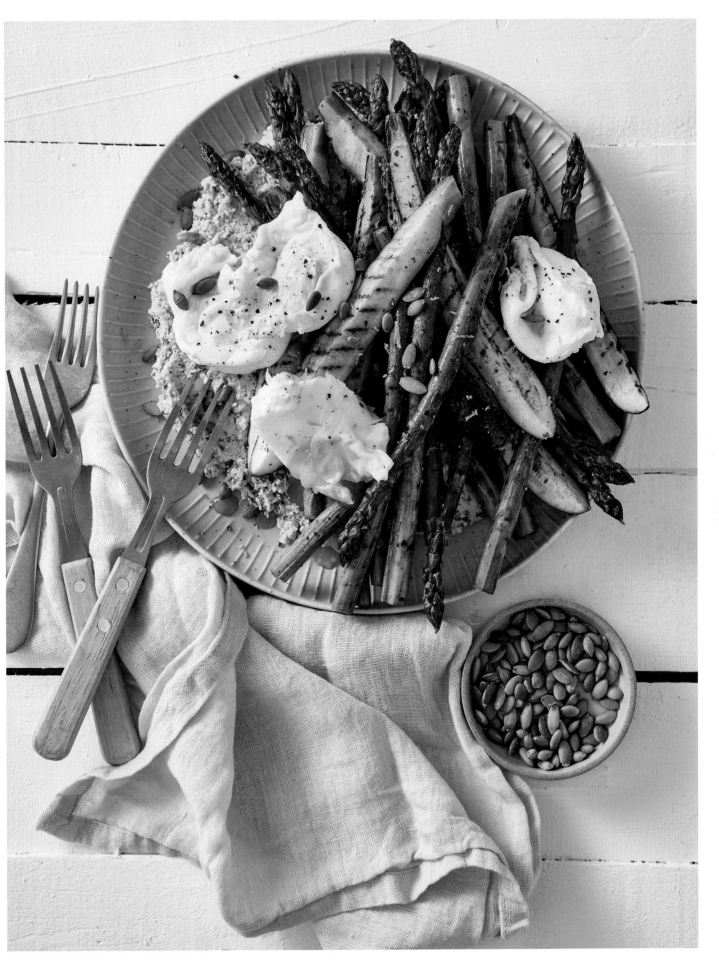

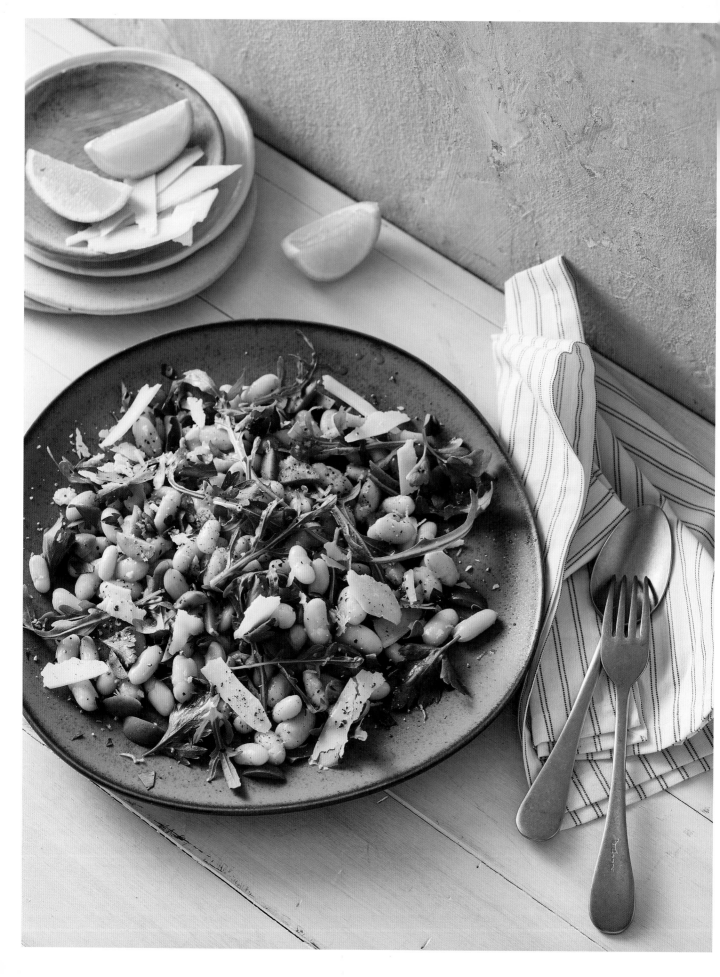

Gremolata beans

🍴 Serves 4   🕐 Preparation: 15 minutes, plus 15 minutes standing time
👨‍🍳 Difficulty: Low

400 g drained, rinsed tinned
cannellini beans (see note)
¼ cup finely chopped flat-leaf parsley
160 g pitted green Sicilian olives,
finely chopped
1 small clove garlic, crushed
Finely grated zest and juice of
1 small lemon
40 g baby rocket leaves
80 g parmesan, shaved

Combine the beans, parsley, olives, garlic, lemon zest and juice together in a bowl and season with freshly ground black pepper. Stand at room temperature, tossing occasionally, for 15 minutes to macerate.

Divide the bean mixture among plates, top with the rocket leaves and sprinkle with the parmesan shavings to serve.

Note: You will require 2 x 400 g tins of cannellini beans for this recipe. Store any leftover beans in an airtight container in the fridge for up to 3 days.

UNITS PER SERVE

BREADS, CEREALS, LEGUMES, STARCHY VEGETABLES	DAIRY	LEAN MEAT, FISH, POULTRY, EGGS, TOFU	LOW-CARB VEGETABLES	MODERATE-CARB VEGETABLES	HEALTHY FATS
1	1	0	1	0	2

Curried frying-pan eggs

GRAMS CARB

13

PER SERVE

🍽 Serves 4   🕐 Preparation: 10 minutes
🍲 Cooking: 15 minutes   👨‍🍳 Difficulty: Medium

WEEKEND FOOD

2 tablespoons korma curry paste

2 x 400 g tins diced tomatoes

1 bunch broccolini, trimmed
and chopped

2 bunches asparagus, trimmed
and chopped

160 g drained, rinsed tinned
lentils (see note)

4 x 55 g eggs

80 g Danish feta, crumbled

¼ cup chopped flat-leaf parsley

Heat a large deep non-stick frying pan over medium–high heat. Add the curry paste and tomatoes and cook, stirring occasionally, for 5 minutes or until slightly thickened.

Add the broccolini and asparagus. Cover and cook, untouched, for 3 minutes, then remove the lid and stir through the lentils. Cook, stirring, for 1 minute.

Using a large spoon, make four deep indents in the tomato mixture, then crack an egg into each one. Cook, partially covered, for 5 minutes or until the egg whites are set and the yolks are still runny.

Remove the pan from the heat and sprinkle the feta and parsley over the top. Take the pan to the table and serve.

Note: You will require 1 x 400 g tin of lentils for this recipe. Store any leftover lentils in an airtight container in the fridge for up to 3 days.

UNITS PER SERVE

BREADS, CEREALS, LEGUMES, STARCHY VEGETABLES	DAIRY	LEAN MEAT, FISH, POULTRY, EGGS, TOFU	LOW-CARB VEGETABLES	MODERATE-CARB VEGETABLES	HEALTHY FATS
0.5	1	0.5	1.5	0	2

Couscous scramble

GRAMS CARB
19
PER SERVE

🍽 Serves 4   🕐 Preparation: 15 minutes, plus 10 minutes standing time
〰 Cooking: 5 minutes   🎓 Difficulty: Low

80 g wholemeal couscous
1 teaspoon dried mixed herbs
¾ cup (180 ml) salt-reduced chicken
    stock, heated
100 g baby spinach leaves
250 g cherry tomatoes, quartered
½ cup chopped flat-leaf parsley
1 tablespoon olive oil margarine
4 x 55 g eggs, whisked
40 g toasted unsalted pistachio
    kernels, chopped
80 g aged cheddar, crumbled
Lemon wedges, to serve

Combine the couscous, dried herbs and hot stock in a heatproof bowl. Cover and stand, untouched, for 5–8 minutes or until all the stock has been absorbed and the couscous is tender. Fluff up the grains with a fork. Add the spinach, tomato and parsley, season with freshly ground black pepper and toss to combine.

Meanwhile, melt the margarine in a large non-stick frying pan over medium heat. Add the egg and cook, stirring occasionally, for 3–4 minutes or until softly set.

Add the scramble egg to the couscous mixture and gently toss to combine. Divide among serving bowls and sprinkle with the pistachios and cheddar. Serve with the lemon wedges.

UNITS PER SERVE

BREADS, CEREALS, LEGUMES, STARCHY VEGETABLES	DAIRY	LEAN MEAT, FISH, POULTRY, EGGS, TOFU	LOW-CARB VEGETABLES	MODERATE-CARB VEGETABLES	HEALTHY FATS
1	1	0.5	1	0	2

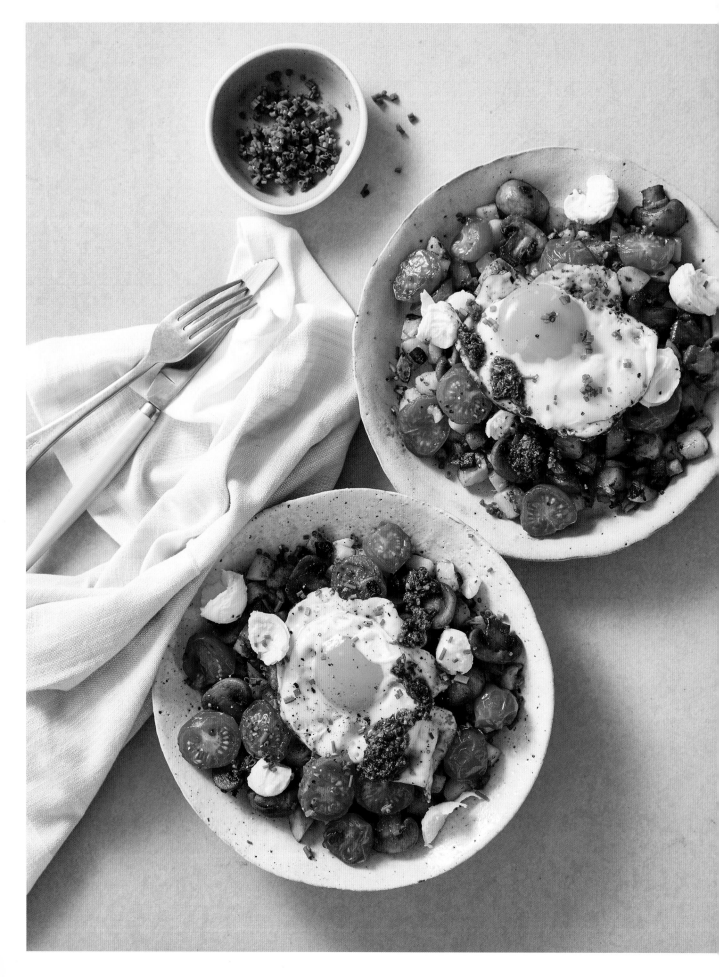

Vegetable hash *and* fried eggs

GRAMS CARB
15
PER SERVE

🍴 **Serves 4**   🕐 **Preparation: 15 minutes**
📚 **Cooking: 15 minutes**   👨‍🍳 **Difficulty: Low**

Olive oil cooking spray
400 g washed kestrel potatoes,
   skin on, cut into 2 cm pieces
200 g small button mushrooms,
   wiped clean and halved
2 zucchini, chopped
250 g cherry tomatoes, halved
2 tablespoons finely chopped chives
100 g baby bocconcini, sliced
4 x 55 g eggs
2 tablespoons basil pesto

Lightly spray a large non-stick frying pan with the oil and place over high heat. Add the potato, mushroom and zucchini and cook, stirring occasionally, for 10 minutes or until golden and almost tender. Reduce the heat to medium. Add the tomatoes and chives and cook, stirring occasionally, for 5 minutes or until softened and golden. Remove the pan from the heat and scatter over the bocconcini. Set aside and allow to melt slightly into the vegetable hash.

Meanwhile, heat another large non-stick frying pan over high heat. Crack the eggs into the pan and cook, untouched, for 3–4 minutes or until the whites are set firm with crispy edges and the yolks are still runny.

Divide the vegetable hash among plates and top with a fried egg. Serve drizzled with the pesto.

UNITS PER SERVE

BREADS, CEREALS, LEGUMES, STARCHY VEGETABLES	DAIRY	LEAN MEAT, FISH, POULTRY, EGGS, TOFU	LOW-CARB VEGETABLES	MODERATE-CARB VEGETABLES	HEALTHY FATS
1	1	0.5	2	0	2

Baked stuffed mushrooms

GRAMS CARB
12
PER SERVE

🍴 Serves 4   🕐 Preparation: 20 minutes
🍲 Cooking: 15 minutes   🍳 Difficulty: Low

MAKE AHEAD   **PORTABLE**

100 g baby spinach leaves
Boiling water, for blanching
4 large field mushrooms, wiped clean,
   stems removed and finely chopped
200 g drained, rinsed tinned
   four-bean mix (see note)
80 g Swiss cheese, finely grated
⅓ cup (40 g) basil pesto
Basil leaves, to serve (optional)

Preheat the oven to 200°C (180°C fan-forced) and line a large baking tray with baking paper.

Place the spinach in a large colander in the sink and pour over the boiling water until it has wilted. Cool and refresh under cold running water, then squeeze dry.

Place the mushrooms, cup side up, on the prepared tray. Fill the cavities with the spinach, then the chopped mushroom stems and bean mix. Sprinkle with the cheese.

Bake for 12–15 minutes or until the mushrooms are just cooked and the tops are golden. Drizzle over the pesto, then serve.

Notes: You will require 1 x 400 g tin of four-bean mix for this recipe. Store any leftover beans in an airtight container in the fridge for up to 3 days.

▶ If making ahead, store the cooled baked mushrooms in an airtight container in the fridge for up to 3 days. Serve cold or warm through in the oven at 150°C (130°C fan-forced).

▶ To make it portable, store the mushrooms in airtight containers. Keep cool while transporting.

UNITS PER SERVE

BREADS, CEREALS, LEGUMES, STARCHY VEGETABLES	DAIRY	LEAN MEAT, FISH, POULTRY, EGGS, TOFU	LOW-CARB VEGETABLES	MODERATE-CARB VEGETABLES	HEALTHY FATS
0.5	1	0	1	0	2

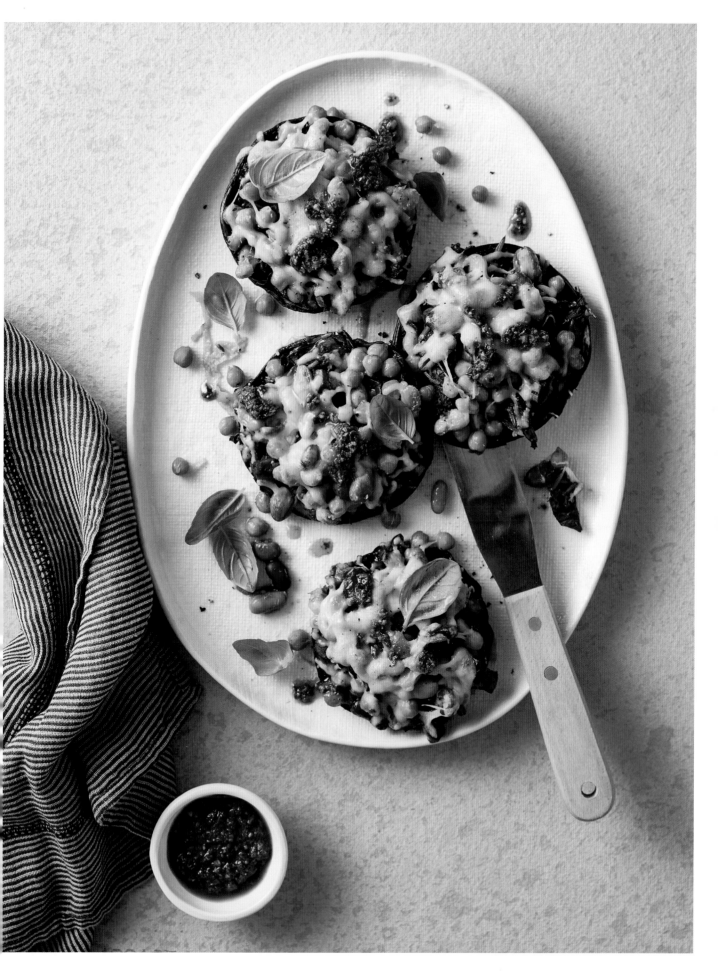

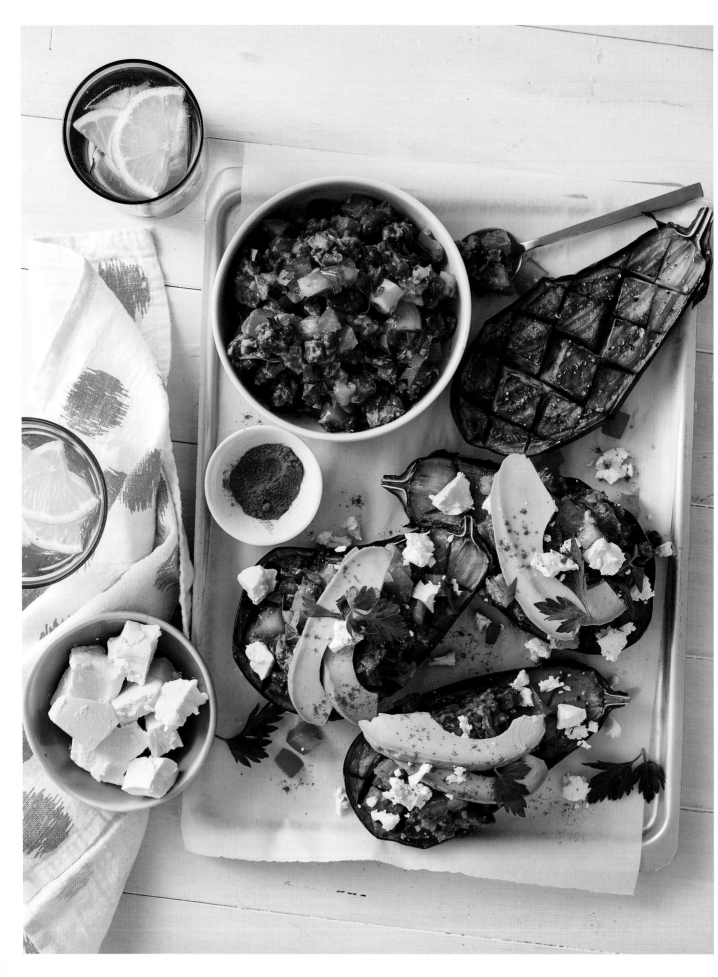

Eggplant subs *with* smashed beans

GRAMS CARB
8
PER SERVE

🍴 Serves 4   🕐 Preparation: 20 minutes
♨ Cooking: 25 minutes   👨‍🍳 Difficulty: Low

2 small eggplants, halved lengthways,
   cut sides scored
Olive oil spray, for cooking
320 g drained, rinsed tinned
   red kidney beans (see note)
2 tablespoons red wine vinegar
1 tablespoon extra virgin olive oil
2 teaspoons sweet paprika
2 tomatoes, finely chopped
¼ cup chopped flat-leaf parsley
80 g avocado, sliced
80 g Danish feta, crumbled

Preheat the oven to 200°C (180°C fan-forced) and line a large baking tray with baking paper.

Place the eggplant, cut side up, on the prepared tray and lightly spray with the olive oil. Season with freshly ground black pepper. Bake for 20–25 minutes or until softened and golden. Transfer to a serving platter.

Meanwhile, place the kidney beans, vinegar, extra virgin olive oil and paprika in a large bowl and lightly mash together. Season with freshly ground black pepper and stir in the tomato.

Just before serving, add the parsley to the bean mixture and gently mix to combine. Spoon evenly over the eggplant halves, scatter over the avocado and feta, and serve.

Note: You will require 2 x 400 g tins of red kidney beans for this recipe. Store any leftover beans in an airtight container in the fridge for up to 3 days.

UNITS PER SERVE

BREADS, CEREALS, LEGUMES, STARCHY VEGETABLES	DAIRY	LEAN MEAT, FISH, POULTRY, EGGS, TOFU	LOW-CARB VEGETABLES	MODERATE-CARB VEGETABLES	HEALTHY FATS
1	1	0	0	1	2

2

LUNCH

Hearty tuna couscous salad

🍴 Serves 4   🕐 Preparation: 25 minutes, plus 10 minutes standing time
👨‍🍳 Difficulty: Low

80 g wholemeal couscous
300 g thawed, peeled broad beans
1 cup (250 ml) salt-reduced chicken
  stock, heated
400 g drained tinned tuna in spring
  water, thickly flaked (see note)
150 g baby radishes, very thinly sliced
  into rounds
4 Lebanese cucumbers, chopped
150 g mixed salad leaves
80 g toasted pecans, halved
80 g Greek feta, finely chopped

MUSTARD DRESSING
2 teaspoons Dijon mustard
Finely grated zest and juice of
  1 large lemon
1 tablespoon extra virgin olive oil

To make the mustard dressing, whisk together all the ingredients and season with freshly ground black pepper. Set aside until you are ready to serve.

Combine the couscous, broad beans and hot stock in a large heatproof bowl. Cover and stand, untouched, for 5–10 minutes or until all the stock has been absorbed and the couscous is tender. Fluff up the grains with a fork.

Add the remaining ingredients to the couscous mixture and toss together well. Divide among plates, drizzle with the mustard dressing and serve.

Note: You will require 1 x 425 g tin of tuna for this recipe. Store the leftover tuna in an airtight container in the fridge for up to 3 days.

UNITS PER SERVE

BREADS, CEREALS, LEGUMES, STARCHY VEGETABLES	DAIRY	LEAN MEAT, FISH, POULTRY, EGGS, TOFU	LOW-CARB VEGETABLES	MODERATE-CARB VEGETABLES	HEALTHY FATS
1	1	1	2	1	3

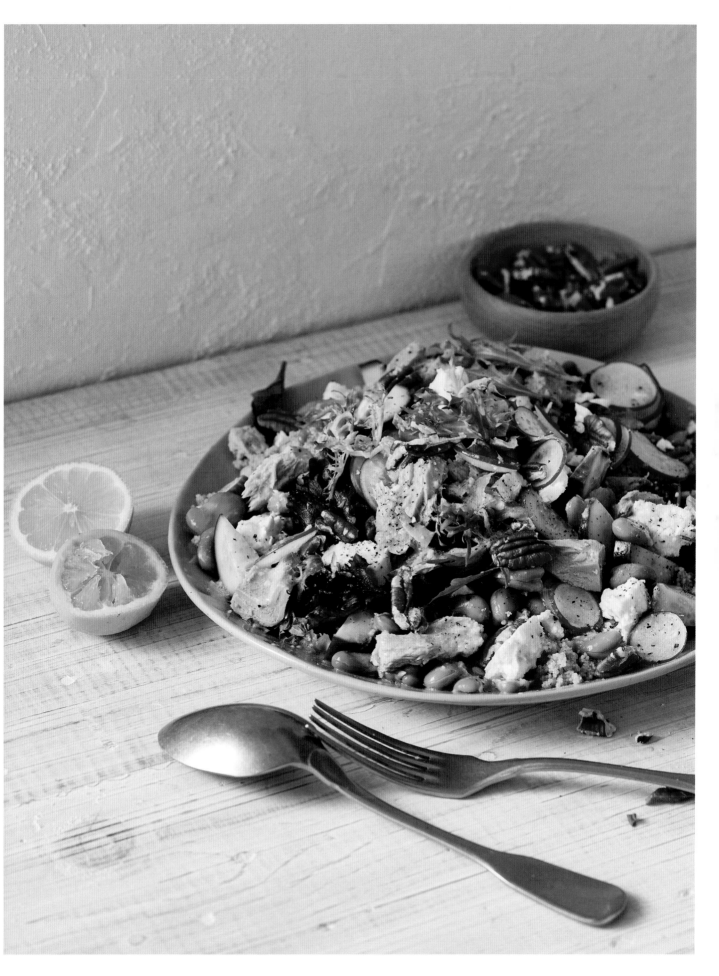

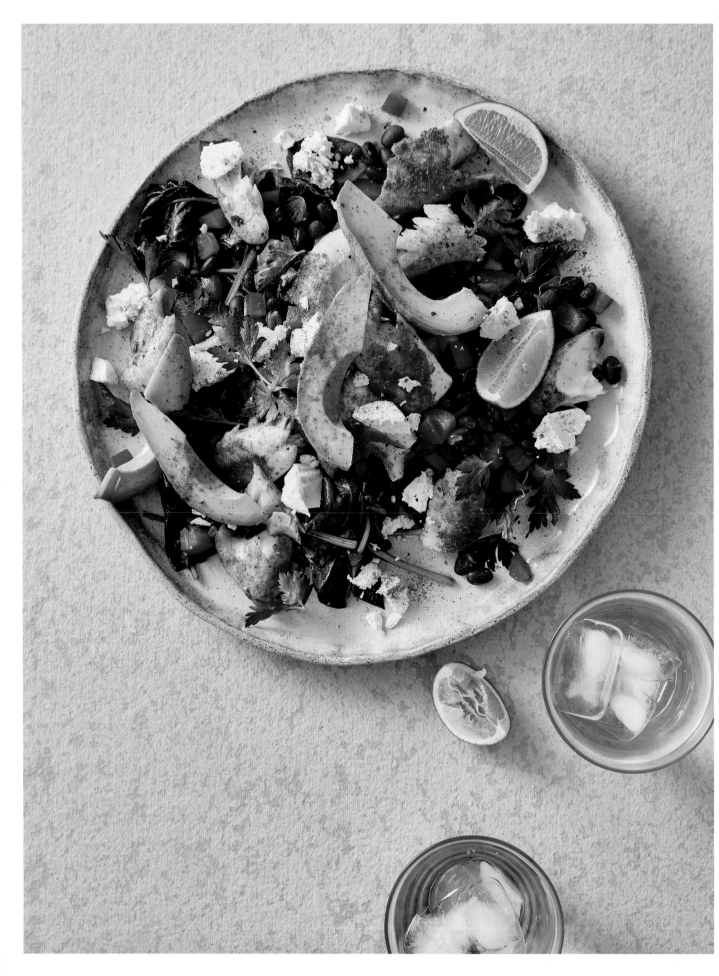

Mexican fish and black beans

GRAMS CARB
11
PER SERVE

🍴 **Serves 4** 🕐 **Preparation: 25 minutes**
🍲 **Cooking: 10 minutes** 🍳 **Difficulty: Low**

200 g drained, rinsed tinned
   black beans (see note)
160 g avocado, sliced
1 red capsicum, seeded and
   finely chopped
½ cup flat-leaf parsley leaves
Finely grated zest and juice of 2 limes,
   plus lime wedges to serve
200 g skinless, boneless
   flathead fillets
3 teaspoons Mexican seasoning
1 tablespoon olive oil
300 g baby spinach leaves
80 g Danish feta, crumbled

Combine the black beans, avocado, capsicum, parsley, lime zest and juice in a bowl and season with freshly ground black pepper. Set aside at room temperature.

Coat the fish evenly in the seasoning. Heat the oil in a large non-stick frying pan over high heat. Add the fish and cook, turning occasionally, for 6–8 minutes or until just cooked and golden. Transfer to a board and thickly flake.

Add the spinach and 1 tablespoon water to the pan and cook, tossing, for 1 minute or until just wilted.

Divide the spinach among plates. Top with the black bean mixture, then the fish. Sprinkle with the feta and serve with the lime wedges.

Note: You will require 1 x 400 g tin of black beans for this recipe. Store any leftover beans in an airtight container in the fridge for up to 3 days.

UNITS PER SERVE

BREADS, CEREALS, LEGUMES, STARCHY VEGETABLES	DAIRY	LEAN MEAT, FISH, POULTRY, EGGS, TOFU	LOW-CARB VEGETABLES	MODERATE-CARB VEGETABLES	HEALTHY FATS
0.5	1	0.5	2	0.5	3

Salmon salad *with* seasoned toast

GRAMS CARB
17
PER SERVE

🍴 Serves 4   🕐 Preparation: 25 minutes
🍳 Cooking: 5 minutes   👨‍🍳 Difficulty: Low

2 tablespoons extra virgin olive oil
2 tablespoons red wine vinegar
400 g drained tinned red salmon, flaked (see note)
150 g baby spinach leaves
150 g baby rocket leaves
300 g red cabbage, very finely shredded
2 Lebanese cucumbers, peeled into long, thin ribbons
1 carrot, peeled into thin ribbons
2 spring onions, thinly sliced
80 g parmesan, shaved

SEASONED TOAST
Olive oil spray, for cooking
4 x 35 g slices multigrain bread
2 teaspoons salt-reduced garlic and herb seasoning

To make the seasoned toast, preheat the oven grill to high. Lightly spray the bread slices with oil on both sides, then sprinkle evenly with the seasoning. Cook under the grill for 1–2 minutes each side or until golden and crisp. Remove, then cut each slice into three thick fingers. Set aside.

Whisk together the oil and vinegar in a large bowl and season with freshly ground black pepper. Add all the remaining ingredients and gently toss to combine.

Divide the salad among bowls and serve with the seasoned toast.

Note: You will require 1 x 415 g tin of red salmon for this recipe. Store the leftover salmon in an airtight container in the fridge for up to 3 days.

UNITS PER SERVE

BREADS, CEREALS, LEGUMES, STARCHY VEGETABLES	DAIRY	LEAN MEAT, FISH, POULTRY, EGGS, TOFU	LOW-CARB VEGETABLES	MODERATE-CARB VEGETABLES	HEALTHY FATS
1	1	1	2	1	2

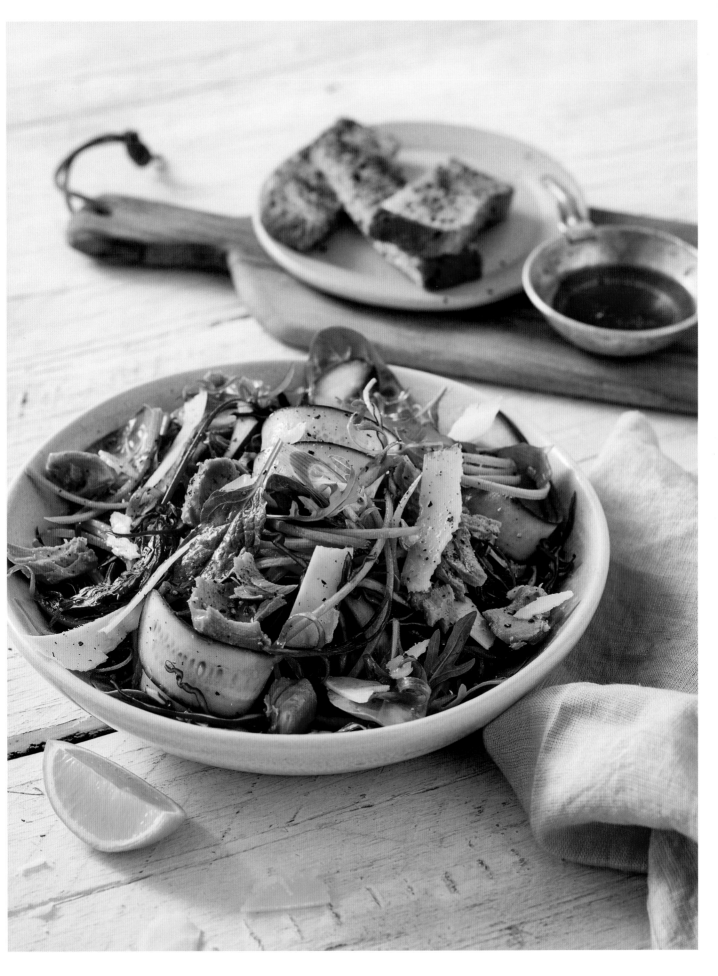

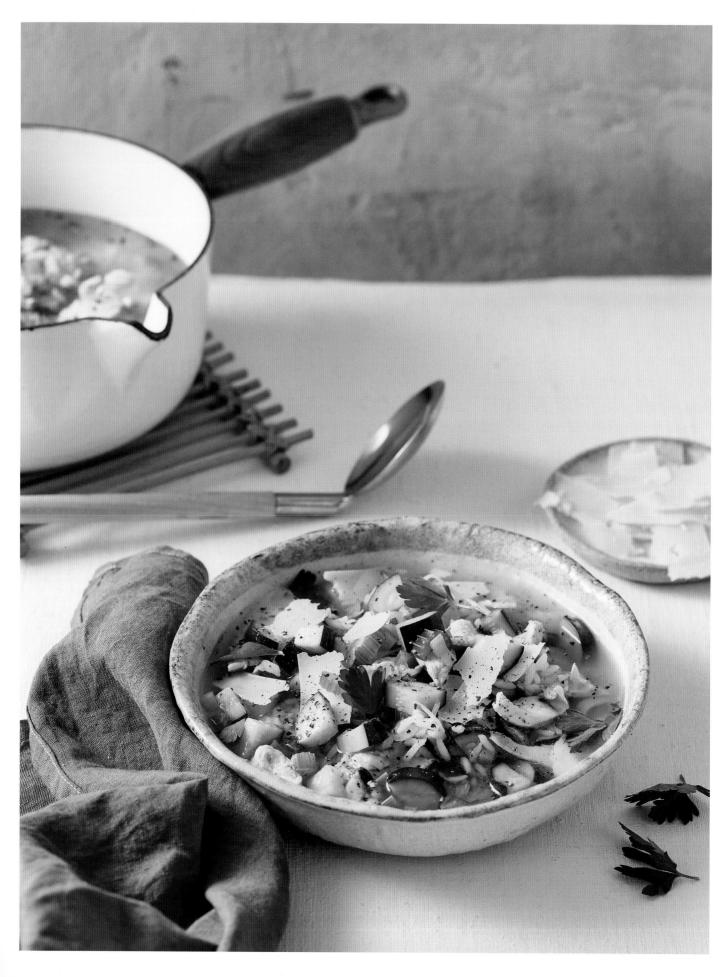

Chicken *and* rice soup

GRAMS CARB 14 PER SERVE

🍴 Serves 4   🕐 Preparation: 20 minutes
🍲 Cooking: 20 minutes   👨‍🍳 Difficulty: Low

80 g low-GI rice
2 tablespoons olive oil
2 cloves garlic, crushed
1 teaspoon dried mixed herbs
1 leek, white part only, thinly sliced
6 sticks celery, thinly sliced
6 small zucchini, chopped
400 g chicken tenderloins,
   thinly sliced
1.5 litres (6 cups) salt-reduced
   chicken stock
¼ cup chopped flat-leaf parsley
80 g parmesan, finely grated

Bring a saucepan of water to the boil over high heat, add the rice and cook for 8–10 minutes or until just tender. Drain, then refresh under cold running water. Drain again.

Meanwhile, heat the oil in a large saucepan over high heat. Add the garlic, mixed herbs, leek, celery and zucchini and cook, stirring occasionally, for 10 minutes or until softened.

Reduce the heat to medium and add the chicken, stock and 500 ml (2 cups) water. Stir well, then simmer for 10 minutes or until the chicken is tender. Remove the pan from the heat. Stir through the cooked rice and season with freshly ground black pepper.

Ladle the soup into bowls, and serve sprinkled with the parsley and parmesan.

UNITS PER SERVE

BREADS, CEREALS, LEGUMES, STARCHY VEGETABLES	DAIRY	LEAN MEAT, FISH, POULTRY, EGGS, TOFU	LOW-CARB VEGETABLES	MODERATE-CARB VEGETABLES	HEALTHY FATS
1	1	1	2	0.5	2

Salmon rice salad *with* basil almond dressing

GRAMS CARB
14
PER SERVE

🍴 Serves 4　　🕐 Preparation: 20 minutes
〰 Cooking: 10 minutes　　👨‍🍳 Difficulty: Low

80 g low-GI rice

4 baby cos lettuces, cut into wedges

1 bunch baby radishes, very thinly
　　sliced into rounds

4 Lebanese cucumbers, chopped

400 g drained tinned red salmon,
　　flaked (see note)

80 g Greek feta, crumbled

BASIL ALMOND DRESSING

½ cup basil leaves

1 small clove garlic

2 tablespoons extra virgin olive oil

¼ cup (60 ml) white wine vinegar

1 tablespoon almond butter (see note)

Bring a saucepan of water to the boil over high heat, add the rice and cook for 8–10 minutes or until just tender. Drain, then refresh under cold running water. Drain again.

Meanwhile, to make the basil almond dressing, place all the ingredients in an upright blender and blitz until smooth. Season with freshly ground black pepper.

Divide the lettuce, radish, cucumber, rice, salmon and feta among bowls. Drizzle with the dressing and serve.

Notes: You will require 1 x 415 g tin of red salmon for this recipe. Store the leftover salmon in an airtight container in the fridge for up to 3 days.

▶ It is important to use a good-quality thick almond butter for this recipe – even better if your local health-food shop grinds fresh nuts into a butter.

UNITS PER SERVE

BREADS, CEREALS, LEGUMES, STARCHY VEGETABLES	DAIRY	LEAN MEAT, FISH, POULTRY, EGGS, TOFU	LOW-CARB VEGETABLES	MODERATE-CARB VEGETABLES	HEALTHY FATS
1	1	1	2	0.5	3

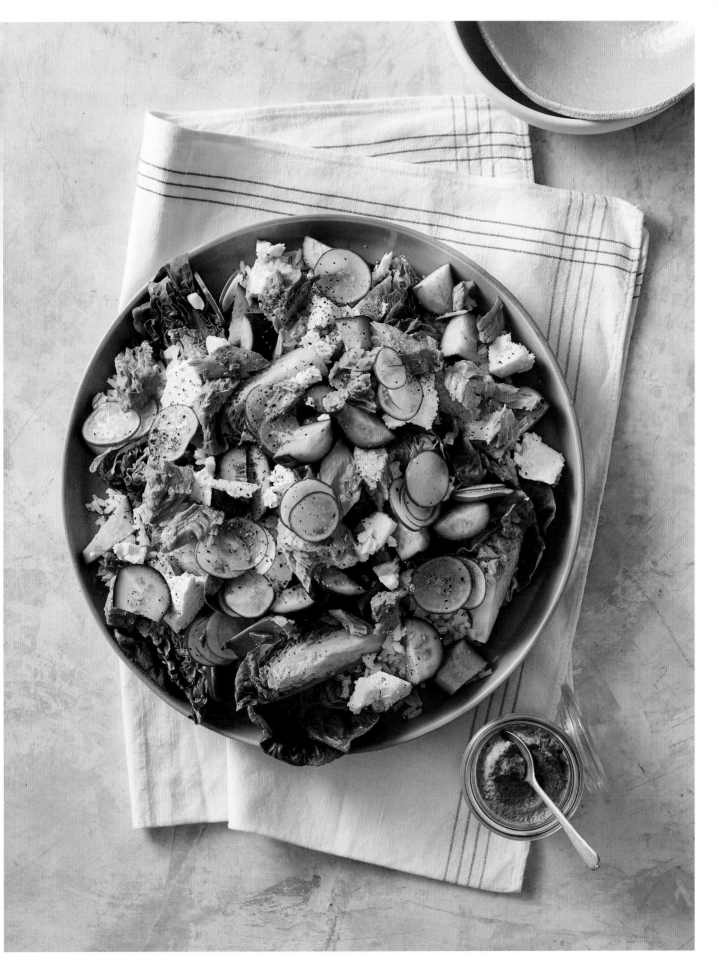

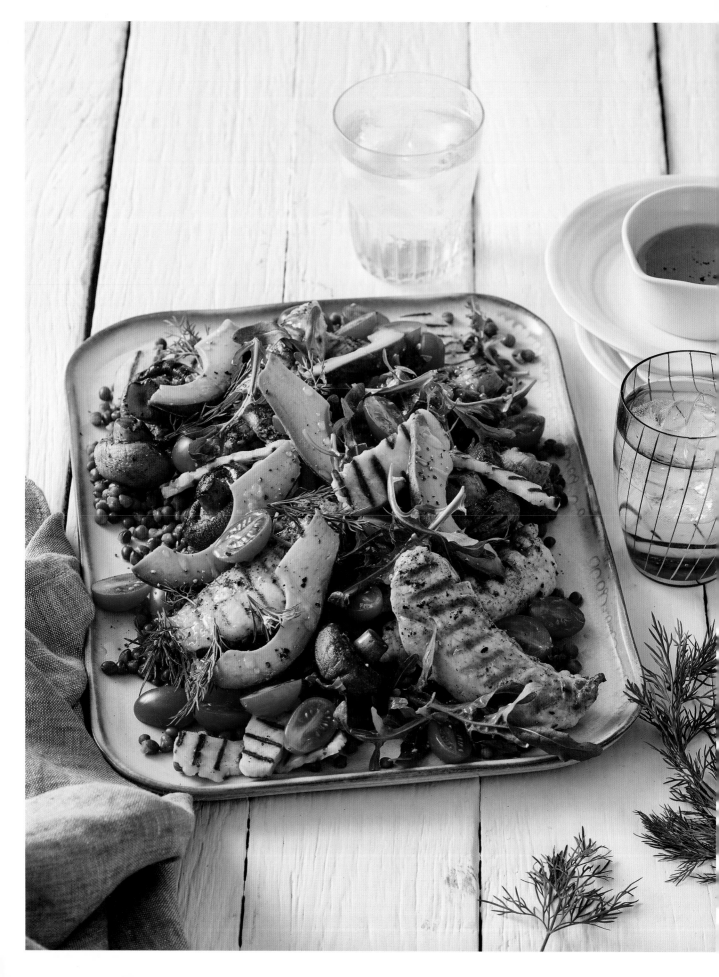

Chargrilled chicken *and* mushrooms *with* avocado lentils

🍴 Serves 4 🕐 Preparation: 20 minutes
〰️ Cooking: 10 minutes 🎩 Difficulty: Low

600 g cup mushrooms, wiped clean
400 g lean chicken tenderloins
80 g haloumi, sliced
360 g drained, rinsed tinned lentils
   (see note)
250 g cherry tomatoes, halved
100 g baby rocket leaves
¼ cup dill fronds
finely grated zest and juice of
   1 large lemon
1 tablespoon extra virgin olive oil
160 g avocado, sliced

Preheat a large chargrill pan over high heat. Season the mushrooms and chicken with freshly ground black pepper, add to the pan and cook, turning occasionally, for 6–8 minutes or until tender and golden. Chargrill the haloumi for 30 seconds each side until warmed through and light golden.

Meanwhile, combine all the remaining ingredients, except the avocado, in a large bowl. Season with freshly ground black pepper.

Divide the lentil mixture among plates and top with the avocado, mushrooms, chicken and haloumi.

Note: You will require 2 x 400 g tins of lentils for this recipe. Store leftover lentils in an airtight container in the fridge for up to 3 days.

UNITS PER SERVE

BREADS, CEREALS, LEGUMES, STARCHY VEGETABLES	DAIRY	LEAN MEAT, FISH, POULTRY, EGGS, TOFU	LOW-CARB VEGETABLES	MODERATE-CARB VEGETABLES	HEALTHY FATS
1	1	1	2	0	3

Spring vegetable *and* chicken noodle soup

GRAMS CARB
20
PER SERVE

🍴 Serves 4 🕐 Preparation: 15 minutes
〰 Cooking: 10 minutes 👨‍🍳 Difficulty: Low

1 litre (4 cups) salt-reduced chicken
  stock
1 leek, white part only, thinly sliced
2 small zucchini, thinly sliced
2 bunches asparagus, trimmed
  and chopped
400 g lean chicken breast fillet,
  finely chopped
120 g dried wholemeal spaghetti,
  broken into smaller pieces
150 g baby spinach leaves
100 g baby bocconcini, torn
2 tablespoons basil pesto

Place the stock, leek, zucchini, asparagus, chicken and spaghetti in a large saucepan over high heat. Bring to the boil, stirring, then reduce the heat to medium and simmer, covered and stirring occasionally, for 5 minutes or until the pasta is al dente.

Remove the pan from the heat. Add the spinach and stir until wilted.

Ladle the soup into bowls, top with the bocconcini and finish with a dollop of basil pesto.

UNITS PER SERVE

BREADS, CEREALS, LEGUMES, STARCHY VEGETABLES	DAIRY	LEAN MEAT, FISH, POULTRY, EGGS, TOFU	LOW-CARB VEGETABLES	MODERATE-CARB VEGETABLES	HEALTHY FATS
1	1	1	2	1	2

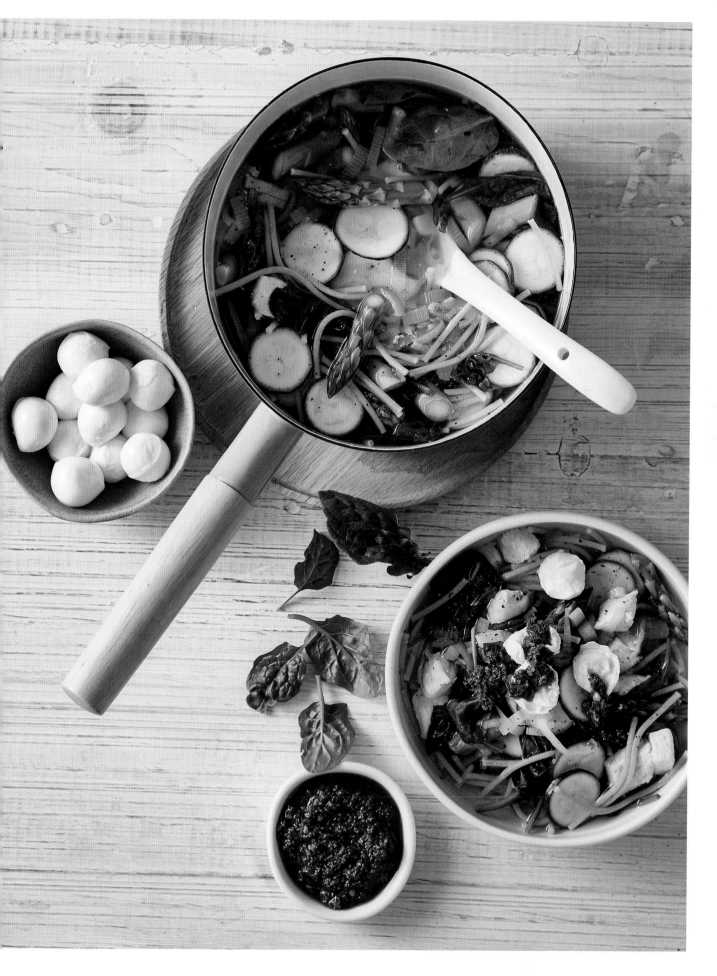

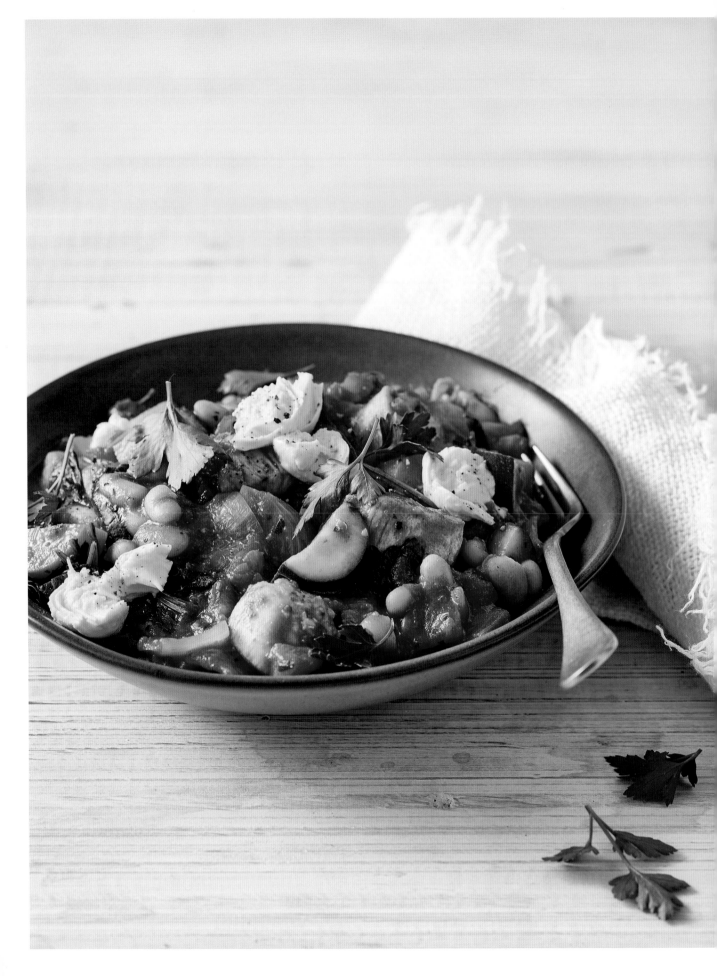

Cannellini bean, chicken *and* vegetable stew

GRAMS CARB
21
PER SERVE

🍴 Serves 4   🕐 Preparation: 20 minutes
♨ Cooking: 15 minutes   🍲 Difficulty: Low

2 tablespoons olive oil
1 onion, chopped
400 g lean chicken breast fillet,
   cut into 1 cm pieces
2 tablespoons fresh Italian herb paste
1 carrot, chopped
4 small zucchini, chopped
2 x 400 g tins chopped tomatoes
400 g drained, rinsed tinned
   cannellini beans (see note)
1 bunch English spinach, leaves picked
1 cup flat-leaf parsley leaves
100 g baby bocconcini, torn
Lemon wedges, to serve (optional)

Heat the oil in a large deep non-stick frying pan over high heat. Add the onion and chicken and cook, stirring occasionally, for 3 minutes.

Add the herb paste, carrot, zucchini, tomatoes and cannellini beans. Reduce the heat to medium and cook, stirring occasionally, for 10 minutes or until the chicken and vegetables are cooked and the sauce has reduced by half. Add the spinach and parsley, stirring until the spinach leaves wilt.

Divide the stew among bowls, top with the bocconcini and serve with the lemon wedges, if desired.

Note: You will require 2 x 400 g tins of cannellini beans for this recipe. Store leftover beans in an airtight container in the fridge for up to 3 days.

UNITS PER SERVE

BREADS, CEREALS, LEGUMES, STARCHY VEGETABLES	DAIRY	LEAN MEAT, FISH, POULTRY, EGGS, TOFU	LOW-CARB VEGETABLES	MODERATE-CARB VEGETABLES	HEALTHY FATS
1	1	1	2	0.5	2

Chargrilled chicken pasta *with* nutty sauce

GRAMS CARB
25
PER SERVE

🍴 Serves 4   🕐 Preparation: 20 minutes
〰 Cooking: 15 minutes   🎩 Difficulty: Low

120 g dried wholemeal spaghetti,
    broken into smaller pieces
500 g fresh zucchini noodles
    (see note)
4 large tomatoes, each sliced into
    3 rounds
1 small red onion, sliced into
    thin rounds
400 g lean chicken breast
    stir-fry strips
80 g parmesan, finely grated

NUTTY SAUCE
160 g toasted mixed unsalted nuts
    (such as pine nuts, almonds,
    pecans), chopped
¼ cup finely chopped mint
½ cup (125 ml) red wine vinegar
2 tablespoons fresh Italian herb paste

To make the nutty sauce, combine all the ingredients in a large bowl.

Cook the pasta in a saucepan of boiling water over high heat for 5 minutes or until al dente. Drain well, then immediately transfer to the bowl with the nutty sauce. Add the zucchini noodles and toss to combine well. Season with freshly ground black pepper.

Meanwhile, heat a large chargrill pan over high heat. Add the tomato and onion and cook, turning occasionally, for 5 minutes or until just tender and golden. Add to the pasta mixture. Chargrill the chicken for 6–8 minutes or until cooked and golden. Add to the pasta mixture and toss everything together.

Divide the pasta mixture among plates, sprinkle with the parmesan and serve warm.

Note: You'll find fresh zucchini noodles in the fresh produce section at the supermarket. If unavailable, you can simply cut 4 zucchini into thin matchsticks and use as directed in the recipe.

UNITS PER SERVE

BREADS, CEREALS, LEGUMES, STARCHY VEGETABLES	DAIRY	LEAN MEAT, FISH, POULTRY, EGGS, TOFU	LOW-CARB VEGETABLES	MODERATE-CARB VEGETABLES	HEALTHY FATS
1	1	1	2	0.5	2

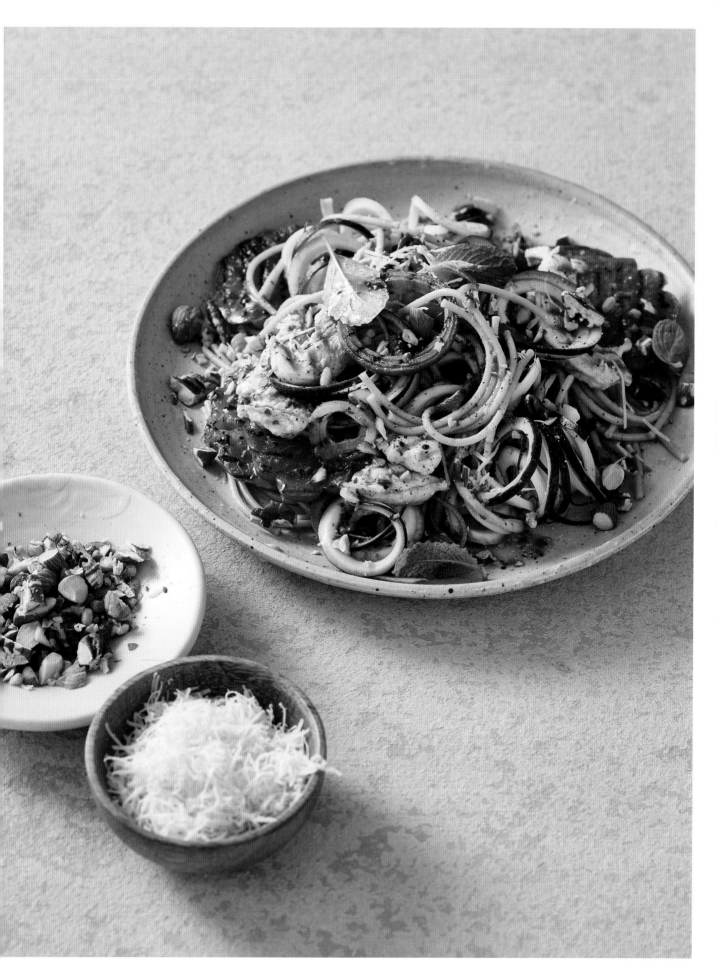

Asparagus *and* salmon spaghetti

GRAMS CARB
25
PER SERVE

🍴 **Serves 4** 🕐 **Preparation: 20 minutes**
🍳 **Cooking: 5 minutes** ⏱ **Difficulty: Low**

120 g dried wholemeal spaghetti,
  broken into thirds
4 bunches asparagus, trimmed and
  cut diagonally into 4 cm lengths
400 g drained tinned red salmon,
  flaked (see note)
120 g baby spinach and rocket leaf mix
200 g mixed baby tomatoes,
  sliced into rounds
1 long red chilli, seeded and
  finely chopped
Finely grated zest and juice of 1 lemon
80 g Danish feta, crumbled
160 g toasted pecans, chopped

Cook the pasta in a saucepan of boiling water over high heat for 4 minutes. Add the asparagus and cook for a further 1 minute or until the pasta is al dente and the asparagus is tender. Drain well and transfer to a large bowl.

Immediately add the salmon, leaf mix, tomato, chilli, lemon zest and juice to the bowl and toss to combine.

Divide the pasta mixture among bowls, sprinkle with the feta and pecans and serve warm.

Note: You will require 1 x 415 g tin of red salmon for this recipe. Store the leftover salmon in an airtight container in the fridge for up to 3 days.

UNITS PER SERVE

BREADS, CEREALS, LEGUMES, STARCHY VEGETABLES	DAIRY	LEAN MEAT, FISH, POULTRY, EGGS, TOFU	LOW-CARB VEGETABLES	MODERATE-CARB VEGETABLES	HEALTHY FATS
1	1	1	2	0	2

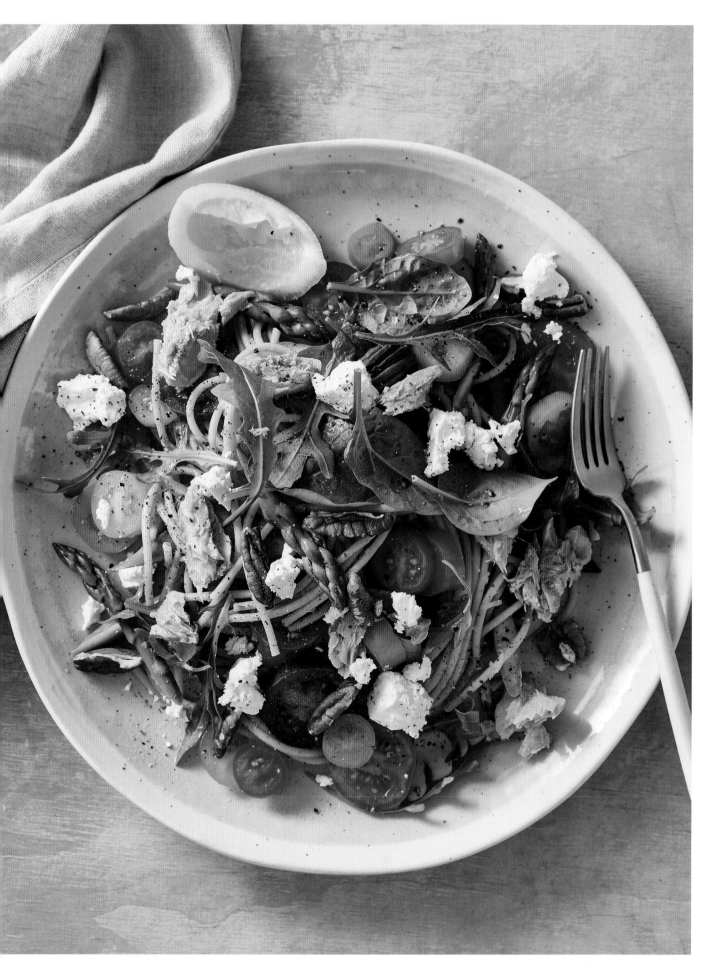

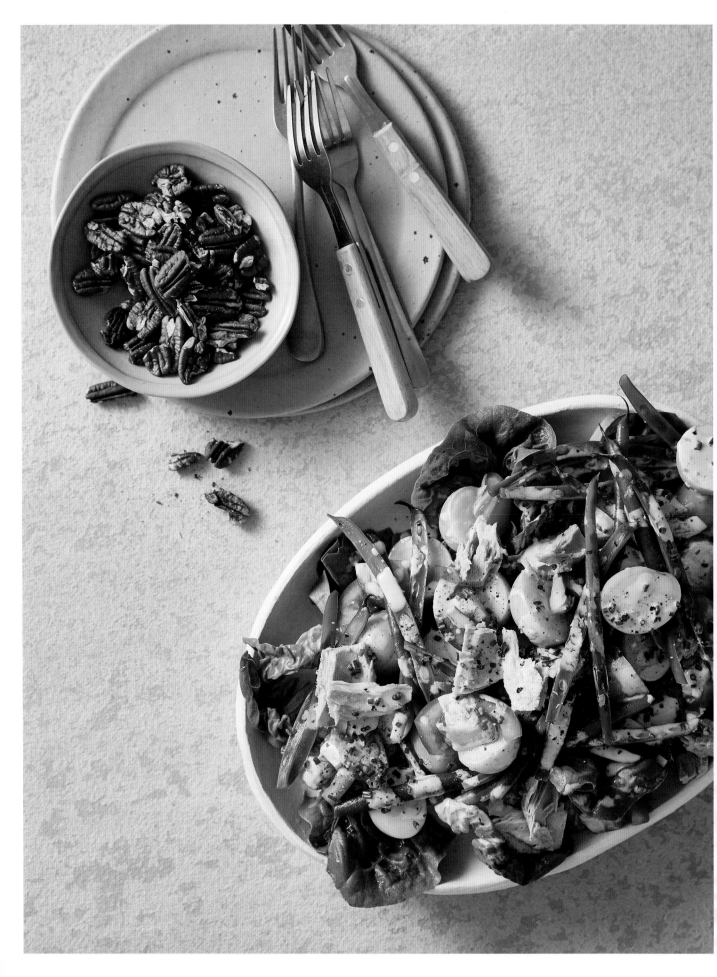

Creamy potato salad *with* tuna

GRAMS CARB
23
PER SERVE

🍴 Serves 4   🕐 Preparation: 25 minutes
🍲 Cooking: 10 minutes   🎓 Difficulty: Low

400 g baby potatoes, halved
300 g baby green beans, trimmed
400 g drained tinned tuna in spring
    water, thickly flaked (see note)
4 roma tomatoes, quartered
    lengthways
4 baby cos lettuces, leaves separated
80 g toasted pecans, chopped

CREAMY DRESSING
400 g Greek-style yoghurt
1 small clove garlic, crushed
1 tablespoon salt-reduced tomato
    paste
1 tablespoon salt-reduced soy sauce
Finely grated zest and juice of
    1 small lemon
1 bunch chives, finely chopped

To make the creamy dressing, mix together all the ingredients in a large bowl and season with freshly ground black pepper. Chill until required.

Cook the potatoes in a saucepan of boiling water over high heat for 8 minutes. Add the beans and cook for a further 2 minutes or until the vegetables are just tender. Drain, then refresh under cold running water. Drain again.

Add the potatoes, beans, tuna and tomato to the dressing and carefully mix to coat and combine.

Divide the cos leaves among plates and top with the potato salad. Sprinkle with the pecans to serve.

Note: You will require 1 x 425 g tin of tuna for this recipe. Store the leftover tuna in an airtight container in the fridge for up to 3 days.

UNITS PER SERVE

BREADS, CEREALS, LEGUMES, STARCHY VEGETABLES	DAIRY	LEAN MEAT, FISH, POULTRY, EGGS, TOFU	LOW-CARB VEGETABLES	MODERATE-CARB VEGETABLES	HEALTHY FATS
1	1	1	2	1	2

Rosemary potato *and* chicken bake

GRAMS CARB
15
PER SERVE

🍴 Serves 4   🕐 Preparation: 20 minutes
🍲 Cooking: 40 minutes   🥘 Difficulty: Low

400 g washed potatoes, very thinly
    sliced into rounds
400 g lean chicken breast stir-fry
    strips
¼ cup rosemary leaves
2 tablespoons olive oil
2 cloves garlic, crushed
2 bulbs baby fennel, cored and thinly
    sliced lengthways
2 bunches broccolini, trimmed
80 g Gruyere cheese, finely grated
2 bunches rocket, trimmed
¼ cup (60 ml) oil-free Italian dressing

Preheat the oven to 220°C (200°C fan-forced).

Place the potato, chicken, rosemary, oil, garlic, fennel and broccolini in two roasting tins and toss to combine and coat well. Season with freshly ground black pepper. Bake, turning occasionally, for 25–30 minutes or until cooked and golden. Sprinkle with the cheese, then bake for a further 10 minutes or until the cheese has melted.

Remove the tins from the oven, add the rocket and dressing and toss to combine. Serve straight from the tins at the table.

UNITS PER SERVE

BREADS, CEREALS, LEGUMES, STARCHY VEGETABLES	DAIRY	LEAN MEAT, FISH, POULTRY, EGGS, TOFU	LOW-CARB VEGETABLES	MODERATE-CARB VEGETABLES	HEALTHY FATS
1	1	1	2	1	2

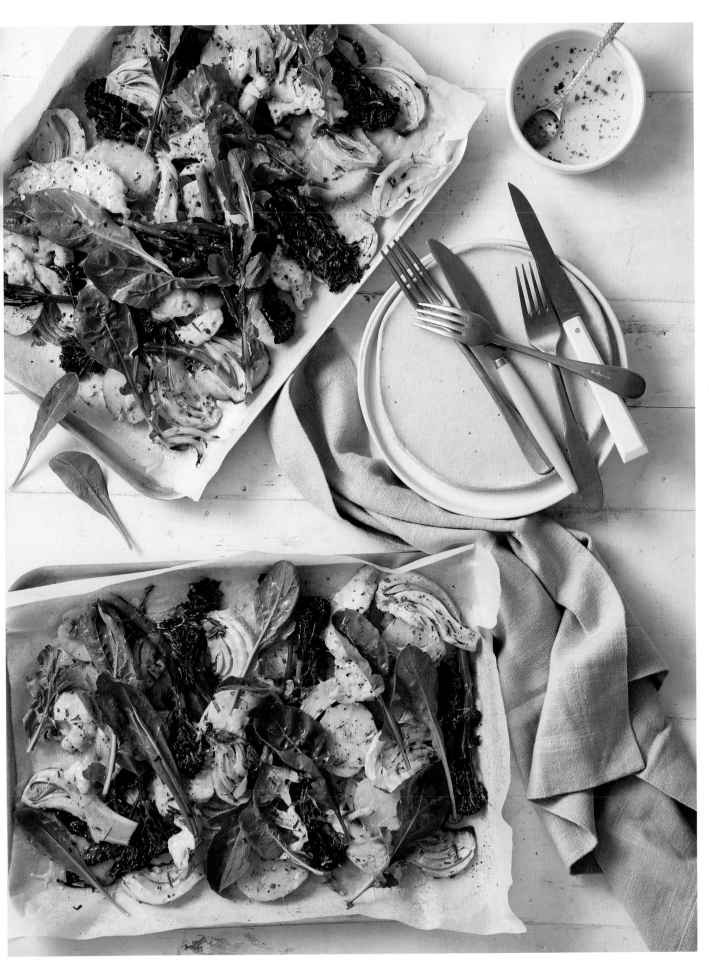

Creamy chicken *and* sweet potato chowder

🍴 Serves 4   🕐 Preparation: 25 minutes
〰 Cooking: 20 minutes   👨‍🍳 Difficulty: Low

1 tablespoon olive oil
1 red onion, finely chopped
2 teaspoons sweet paprika
4 small zucchini, finely chopped
400 g orange sweet potato,
  skin scrubbed, chopped
400 g lean chicken breast fillet,
  finely chopped
1.5 litres (6 cups) salt-reduced
  chicken stock
2 bunches English spinach,
  leaves picked
400 g Greek-style yoghurt
2 tablespoons basil pesto

Heat the oil in a large saucepan over high heat. Add the onion, paprika, zucchini, sweet potato and chicken and cook, stirring occasionally, for 5 minutes or until the onion starts to soften.

Reduce the heat to medium. Add the stock and cook, covered and stirring occasionally, for 15 minutes or until the chicken is cooked and the vegetables are starting to fall apart. Remove the pan from the heat.

Add the spinach leaves and stir until wilted, then stir in the yoghurt. Season with freshly ground black pepper.

Ladle the chowder into bowls, drizzle with the basil pesto and serve.

UNITS PER SERVE

BREADS, CEREALS, LEGUMES, STARCHY VEGETABLES	DAIRY	LEAN MEAT, FISH, POULTRY, EGGS, TOFU	LOW-CARB VEGETABLES	MODERATE-CARB VEGETABLES	HEALTHY FATS
1	1	1	2	0.5	3

Sashimi salmon *with* caper avocado dressing

GRAMS CARB
19
PER SERVE

Serves 4   Preparation: 25 minutes
Difficulty: Low

120 g baby spinach and rocket leaf mix
1 bunch baby radishes, very thinly
  sliced into rounds
2 Lebanese cucumbers, peeled into
  long thin ribbons
4 roma tomatoes, thinly sliced
  into rounds
100 g baby bocconcini, thinly sliced
400 g sashimi-grade salmon,
  very thinly sliced (see note)
Micro herbs, to serve (optional)
8 x 9-Grain Vita-Weats

CAPER AVOCADO DRESSING
1 teaspoon drained, rinsed baby capers
  in vinegar, finely chopped
240 g avocado, finely chopped
2 tablespoons dill fronds
Juice of 1 large lemon

To make the caper avocado dressing, combine all the ingredients in a bowl and season with freshly ground black pepper. Set aside at room temperature.

Divide the leaf mix, radish, cucumber, tomato, bocconcini and salmon among plates. Spoon over the dressing and sprinkle with the micro herbs (if using). Serve with the Vita-Weats alongside.

Note: You can purchase sashimi-grade salmon from reliable fishmongers and ask them to thinly slice it for you.

UNITS PER SERVE					
BREADS, CEREALS, LEGUMES, STARCHY VEGETABLES	DAIRY	LEAN MEAT, FISH, POULTRY, EGGS, TOFU	LOW-CARB VEGETABLES	MODERATE-CARB VEGETABLES	HEALTHY FATS
1	1	1	1	1	4

Curried egg salad *with* mountain bread

🍴 Serves 4   🕐 Preparation: 20 minutes
🍳 Cooking: 5 minutes   👨‍🍳 Difficulty: Low

8 x 55 g eggs
60 g parmesan, shaved
2 wholemeal mountain breads,
    quartered

SALAD
200 g Greek-style yoghurt
Finely grated zest and juice of
    1 large lemon
2 teaspoons curry powder
2 sticks celery, finely chopped
4 Lebanese cucumbers, finely chopped
80 g toasted pine nuts, chopped
150 g baby rocket leaves

Cook the eggs in a saucepan of boiling water for 3–4 minutes for soft-boiled. Drain and cool slightly under cold running water, then peel and cut in half lengthways.

Meanwhile, to make the salad, combine all the ingredients in a bowl. Season with freshly ground black pepper.

Divide the salad among plates and top with the egg halves and parmesan. Serve with the mountain bread.

UNITS PER SERVE

BREADS, CEREALS, LEGUMES, STARCHY VEGETABLES	DAIRY	LEAN MEAT, FISH, POULTRY, EGGS, TOFU	LOW-CARB VEGETABLES	MODERATE-CARB VEGETABLES	HEALTHY FATS
0.5	1	1	1	0	2

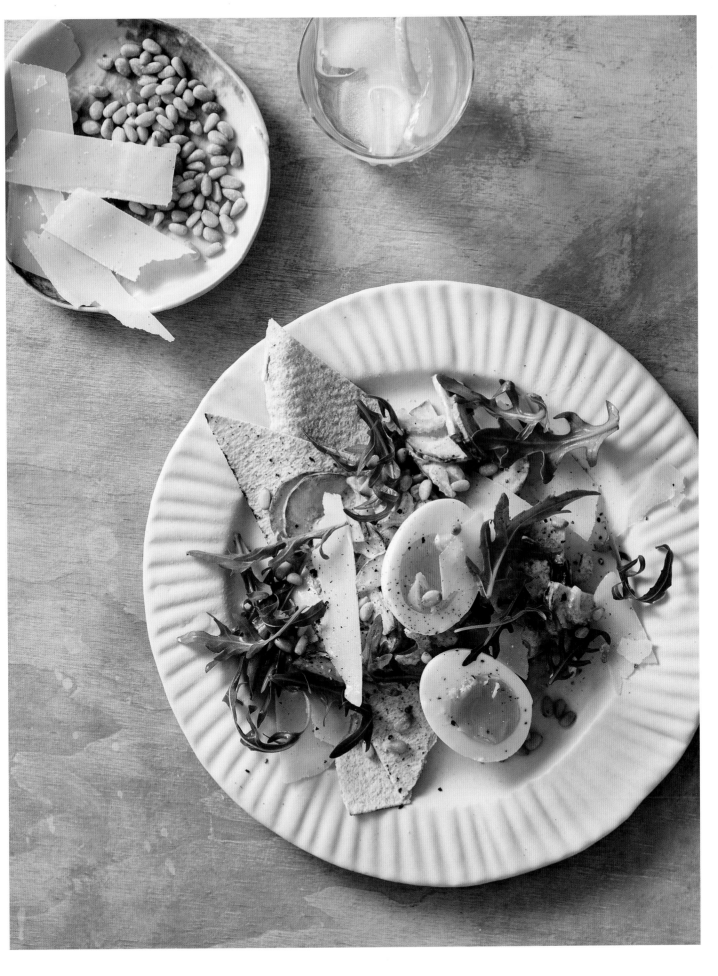

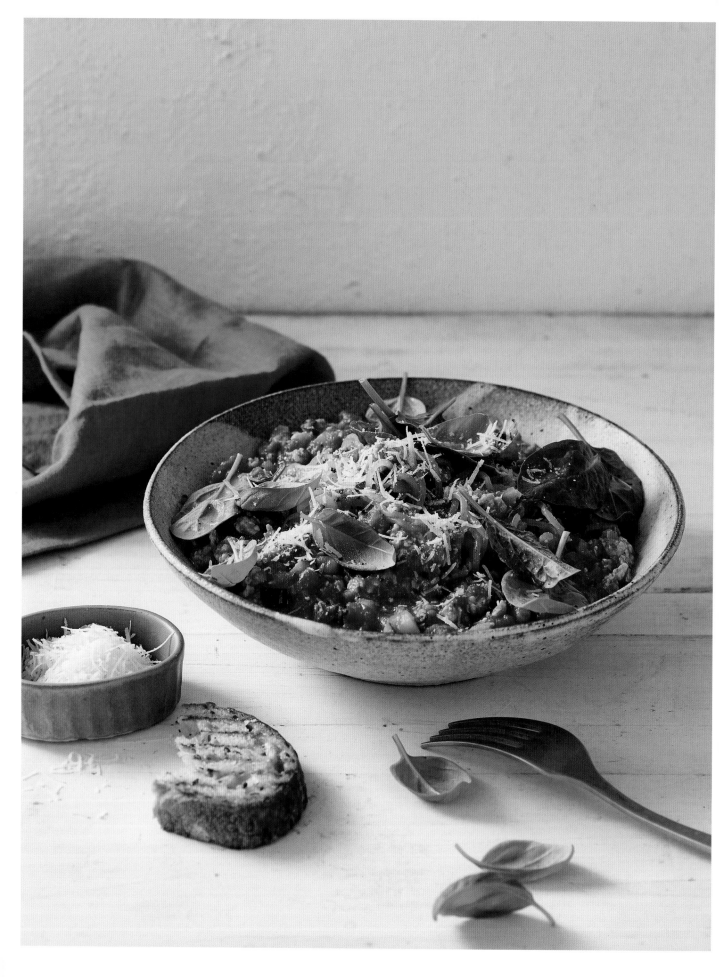

Chicken bolognese
with konjac spaghetti

GRAMS CARB
19
PER SERVE

🍴 **Serves 4**   🕐 **Preparation: 25 minutes**
🍲 **Cooking: 20 minutes**   🎩 **Difficulty: Low**

400 g lean chicken breast fillet, diced
1 tablespoon olive oil
1 onion, finely chopped
4 small zucchini, finely chopped
2 tablespoons fresh Italian herb paste
2 x 400 g tins chopped tomatoes
2 tablespoons salt-reduced
   tomato paste
150 g baby spinach leaves
250 g packet konjac spaghetti,
   drained and rinsed (see note)
1 cup basil leaves
80 g parmesan, finely grated
2 x 35 g slices multigrain bread,
   toasted

Process the chicken in a food processor until finely minced.

Heat the oil in a large deep non-stick frying pan over high heat. Add the onion and zucchini and cook, stirring occasionally, for 3 minutes or until starting to soften. Add the minced chicken and cook, stirring, for 5 minutes, breaking up any large lumps with the back of a spoon.

Reduce the heat to medium. Add the herb paste, tomatoes and tomato paste and cook, stirring occasionally, for 10 minutes or until the sauce has reduced by half. Add the spinach and konjac spaghetti and cook, tossing, for 2 minutes or until the spinach has wilted and the spaghetti is heated through. Season with freshly ground black pepper.

Divide the bolognese among bowls, sprinkle with the basil leaves and parmesan and serve with the toast.

Note: You can find konjac spaghetti in the health-food aisle at the supermarket. It's usually in the gluten-free section.

UNITS PER SERVE

BREADS, CEREALS, LEGUMES, STARCHY VEGETABLES	DAIRY	LEAN MEAT, FISH, POULTRY, EGGS, TOFU	LOW-CARB VEGETABLES	MODERATE-CARB VEGETABLES	HEALTHY FATS
1	1	1	2	0.5	2

Chicken, cashew *and* quinoa toss

GRAMS CARB
21
PER SERVE

🍴 Serves 4   🕐 Preparation: 20 minutes
〰 Cooking: 15 minutes   Difficulty: Low

80 g quinoa, rinsed well and drained
600 g broccoli florets
1 tablespoon olive oil
400 g lean chicken breast
   stir-fry strips
2 tablespoons fresh Italian herb paste
300 g baby green beans, trimmed
½ cup (80 g) toasted unsalted
   cashews, chopped
120 g baby spinach and rocket leaf mix
80 g parmesan, shaved

Cook the quinoa in a saucepan of boiling water for 12–15 minutes or until tender, adding the broccoli to the pan in the last 3 minutes of cooking to lightly steam. Drain.

Meanwhile, heat the oil in a large deep non-stick frying pan over high heat. Add the chicken, herb paste and beans and cook, stirring occasionally, for 2 minutes. Add ¼ cup (60 ml) water and cook, stirring occasionally, for 6–8 minutes or until the chicken is cooked through and lightly golden.

Remove the pan from the heat. Add the cooked quinoa and broccoli, cashews and leaf mix and toss well to combine. Divide among bowls, sprinkle with the parmesan and serve.

UNITS PER SERVE

BREADS, CEREALS, LEGUMES, STARCHY VEGETABLES	DAIRY	LEAN MEAT, FISH, POULTRY, EGGS, TOFU	LOW-CARB VEGETABLES	MODERATE-CARB VEGETABLES	HEALTHY FATS
1	1	1	2	0.5	3

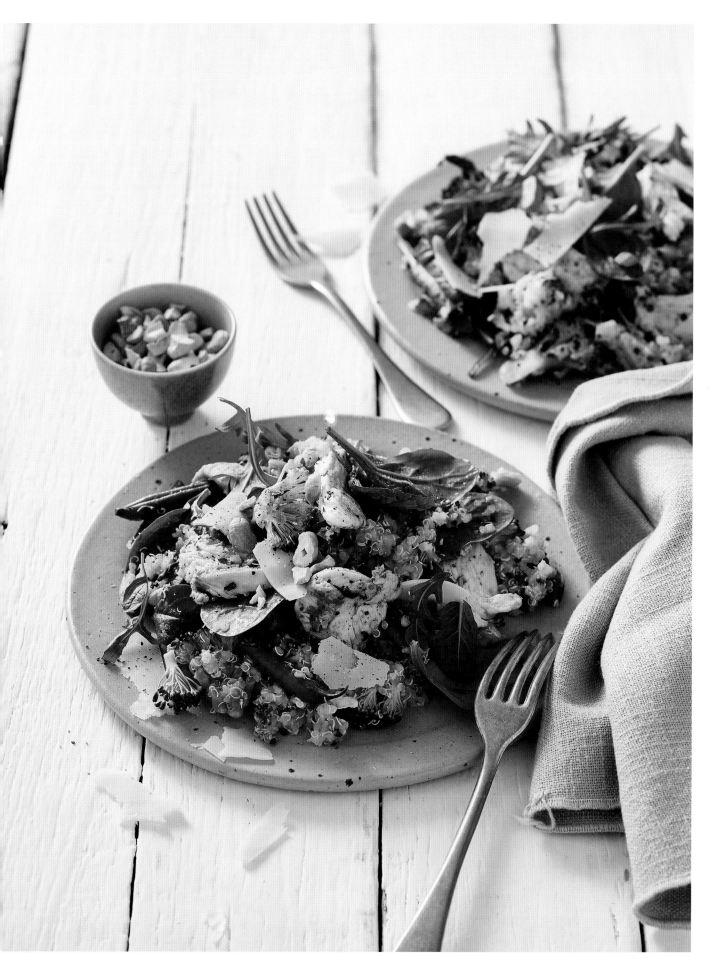

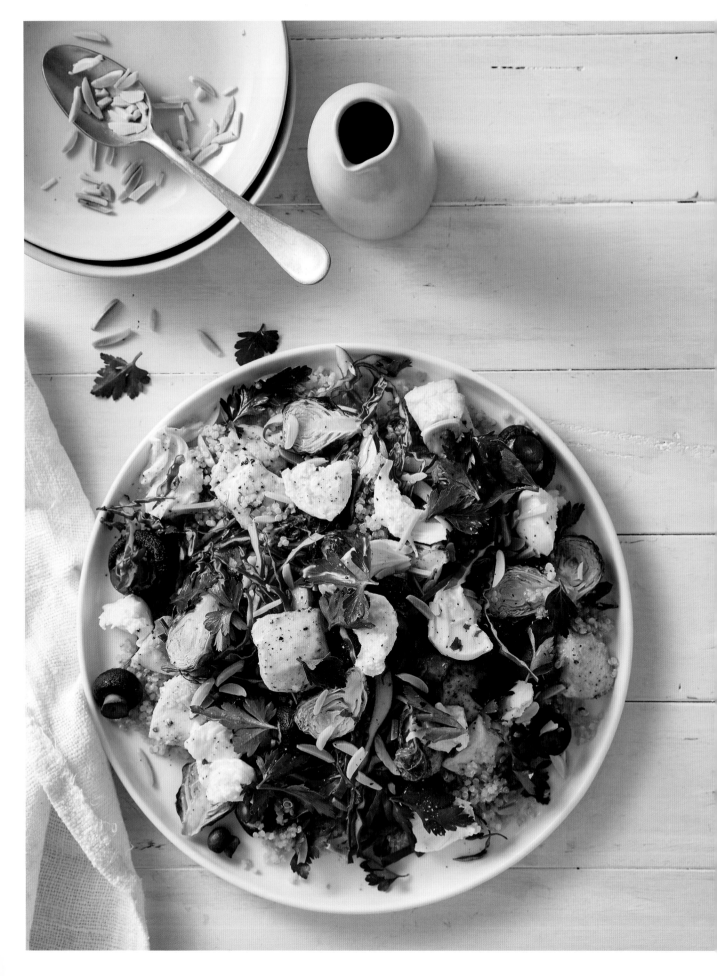

Warm roast chicken, veggie *and* quinoa salad

🍴 Serves 4   🕐 Preparation: 20 minutes
🌀 Cooking: 20 minutes   🎩 Difficulty: Low

GRAMS CARB
16
PER SERVE

400 g lean chicken breast fillet,
cut into 1 cm pieces
150 g brussels sprouts, trimmed
and halved
600 g button mushrooms, wiped clean
80 g slivered almonds
1 tablespoon olive oil
300 g red cabbage, very finely
shredded
80 g quinoa, rinsed well and drained
1 bunch flat-leaf parsley, leaves picked
100 g baby bocconcini, torn
⅓ cup (80 ml) oil-free French dressing

Preheat the oven to 200°C (180°C fan-forced) and line a large baking tray with baking paper.

Add the chicken, brussels sprouts, mushrooms, almonds and oil to the prepared tray and toss well to coat and combine. Roast for 15–20 minutes or until cooked and golden. Transfer to a large bowl, add the cabbage and toss together well.

Meanwhile, cook the quinoa in a saucepan of boiling water for 12–15 minutes or until tender. Drain.

Add the cooked quinoa, parsley, bocconcini and dressing to the chicken mixture and toss to combine. Season with freshly ground black pepper and serve warm.

UNITS PER SERVE

BREADS, CEREALS, LEGUMES, STARCHY VEGETABLES	DAIRY	LEAN MEAT, FISH, POULTRY, EGGS, TOFU	LOW-CARB VEGETABLES	MODERATE-CARB VEGETABLES	HEALTHY FATS
1	1	1	1	1.5	3

Tuna, corn *and* capsicum smash

GRAMS CARB
22
PER SERVE

🍴 Serves 4   🕐 Preparation: 20 minutes
👨‍🍳 Difficulty: Low

400 g drained tinned tuna in
    spring water (see note)
70 g fresh corn kernels
    (from 2 corn cobs)
1 small red capsicum, seeded and
    finely chopped
1 stick celery, finely chopped
2 tablespoons finely chopped chives
1 tablespoon salt-reduced garlic and
    herb seasoning
100 g Greek-style yoghurt
14 rye Cruskits
600 g iceberg lettuce, shredded
60 g Danish feta, crumbled
80 g pine nuts, toasted

Combine the tuna, corn, capsicum, celery, chives, seasoning and yoghurt in a bowl. Season with freshly ground black pepper.

Divide the Cruskits among plates, top with the lettuce, then the tuna smash and the feta and pine nuts to serve.

Note: You will require 1 x 425 g tin of tuna for this recipe. Store the leftover tuna in an airtight container in the fridge for up to 3 days.

UNITS PER SERVE

BREADS, CEREALS, LEGUMES, STARCHY VEGETABLES	DAIRY	LEAN MEAT, FISH, POULTRY, EGGS, TOFU	LOW-CARB VEGETABLES	MODERATE-CARB VEGETABLES	HEALTHY FATS
1	1	1	2	1	2

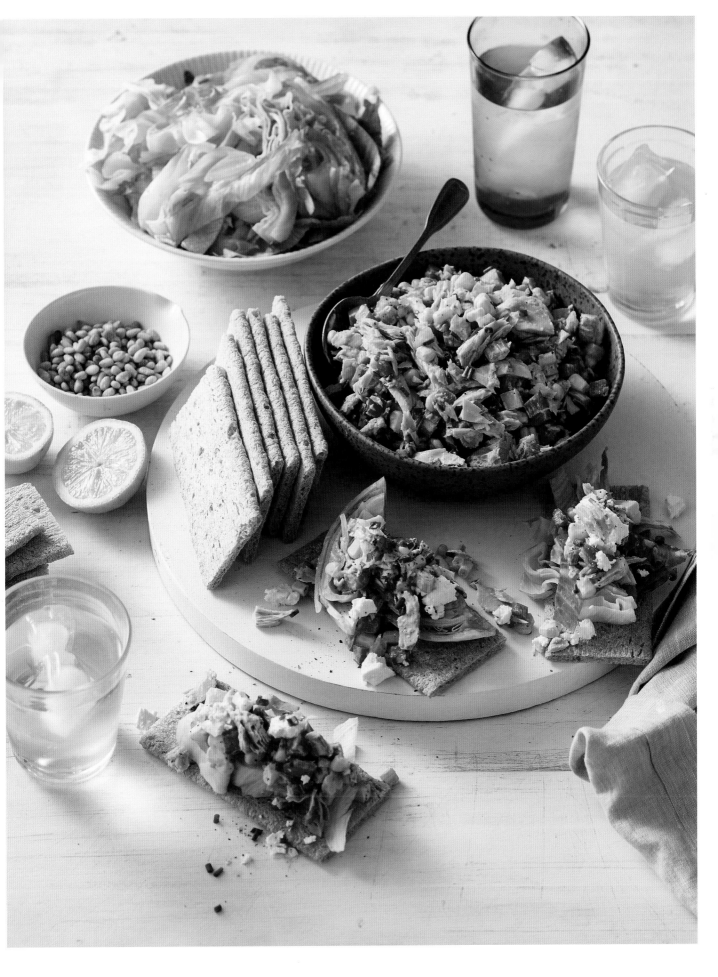

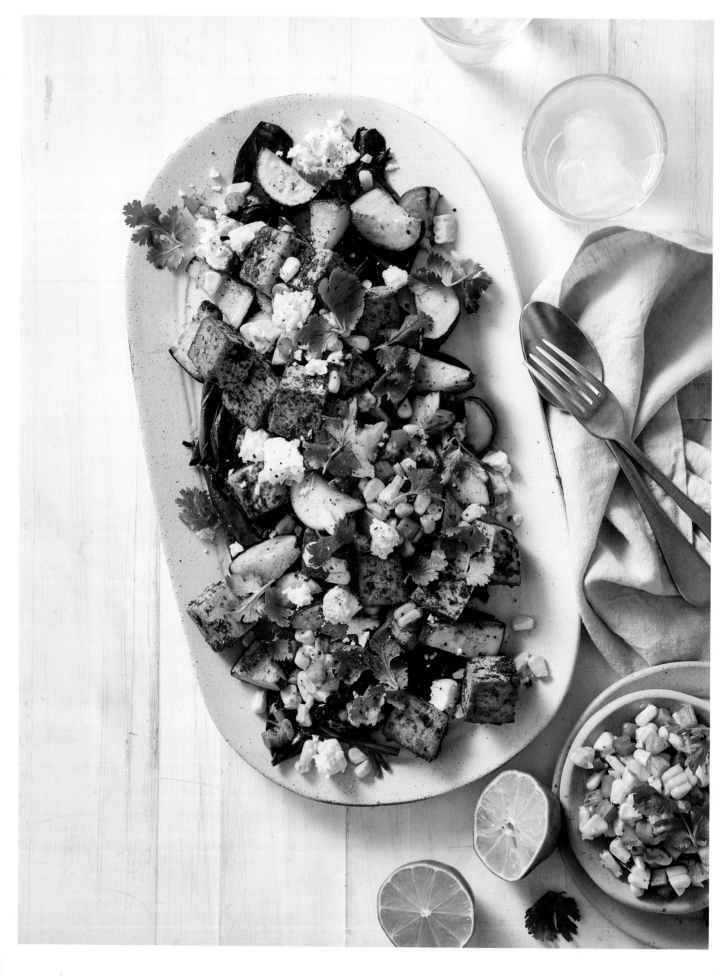

Cajun tofu *with* corn salsa

🍴 Serves 4   🕐 Preparation: 30 minutes
◎ Cooking: 10 minutes   👩‍🍳 Difficulty: Low

1 tablespoon olive oil
200 g firm tofu, patted dry with paper
    towel, cut into 2 cm pieces
1 tablespoon Cajun spice blend
4 zucchini, chopped
2 bunches English spinach,
    leaves picked
80 g Greek feta, crumbled

CORN SALSA
280 g fresh corn kernels
    (from 3 corn cobs)
1 bunch coriander, leaves picked
2 sticks celery, finely chopped
1 tablespoon extra virgin olive oil
Finely grated zest and juice of 2 limes

To make the corn salsa, combine all the ingredients in a bowl and season with freshly ground black pepper. Set aside at room temperature.

Heat the oil in a large deep non-stick frying pan over high heat. Add the tofu and spice blend and cook, tossing, for 1 minute. Add the zucchini and cook, stirring occasionally, for 3 minutes or until starting to soften. Add the spinach and 2 tablespoons water and cook, tossing, for 2 minutes or until wilted.

Divide the tofu mixture among bowls, top with the corn salsa and sprinkle with the feta to serve.

UNITS PER SERVE

BREADS, CEREALS, LEGUMES, STARCHY VEGETABLES	DAIRY	LEAN MEAT, FISH, POULTRY, EGGS, TOFU	LOW-CARB VEGETABLES	MODERATE-CARB VEGETABLES	HEALTHY FATS
1	1	0.5	2	0.5	2

3

POULTRY & PORK DINNERS

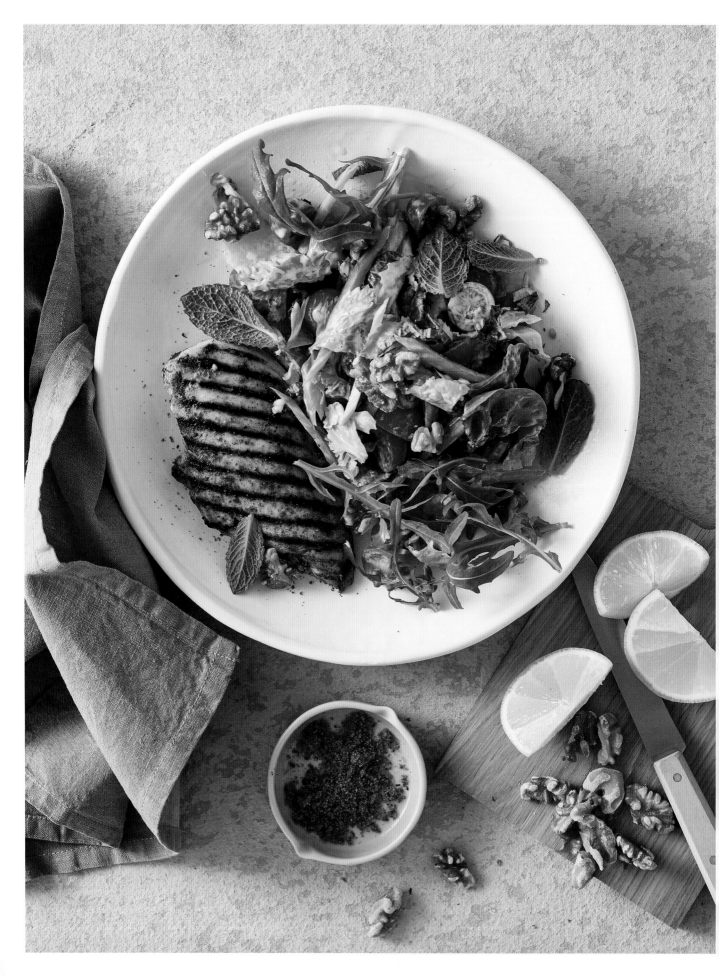

Chargrilled chicken *with* celery salad

GRAMS CARB
5
PER SERVE

🍴 Serves 4　🕐 Preparation: 25 minutes, plus 5 minutes resting time
〰 Cooking: 15 minutes　👨‍🍳 Difficulty: Low

1 tablespoon olive oil
4 x 150 g lean chicken breast fillets
1 tablespoon peri peri spice blend
150 g baby rocket leaves

CELERY SALAD
100 g Greek-style yoghurt
1 small clove garlic, crushed
Finely grated zest and juice of 1 lemon
⅓ cup mint leaves
250 g cherry tomatoes, quartered
4 sticks celery, very thinly sliced
2 baby cos lettuces, roughly chopped
80 g toasted walnuts, chopped

To make the celery salad, whisk the yoghurt, garlic, lemon zest and juice in a large bowl until well combined. Add all the remaining ingredients, season with freshly ground black pepper and toss to combine.

Preheat a large chargrill pan over medium–high heat. Toss the oil, chicken and seasoning together in a bowl and season with freshly ground black pepper.

Chargrill the chicken, turning occasionally, for 10–12 minutes or until golden and cooked through. Transfer to a board, cover loosely with foil and rest for 5 minutes.

Divide the rocket, celery salad and chicken among plates and serve.

UNITS PER SERVE					
BREADS, CEREALS, LEGUMES, STARCHY VEGETABLES	DAIRY	LEAN MEAT, FISH, POULTRY, EGGS, TOFU	LOW-CARB VEGETABLES	MODERATE-CARB VEGETABLES	HEALTHY FATS
0	>0.5	1.5	3	0	2

Slow-cooker chicken cacciatore *with* cauliflower mash

GRAMS CARB
12
PER SERVE

🍴 Serves 4   🕐 Preparation: 25 minutes
♨ Cooking: 4 hours   👨‍🍳 Difficulty: Low

600 g lean chicken tenderloins
2 x 400 g tins chopped tomatoes
1 tablespoon mixed dried herbs
1 red onion, cut into wedges
300 g button mushrooms, wiped clean
2 zucchini, halved lengthways, then
   thickly sliced
80 g pitted green Sicilian olives

CAULIFLOWER MASH
450 g cauliflower florets
160 g avocado
1 tablespoon olive oil margarine
2 tablespoons finely chopped
   flat-leaf parsley

Set a slow-cooker to high. Add all the ingredients, then cover and cook for 4 hours.

Shortly before the chicken is ready, prepare the cauliflower mash. Steam the cauliflower over a saucepan of boiling water for 12–15 minutes or until tender. Transfer to a bowl, add the avocado, margarine and parsley and mash together. Season with freshly ground black pepper.

Divide the cauliflower mash among bowls, add the chicken cacciatore and serve.

Note: Don't worry if you don't have a slow-cooker – you can also make this on the stovetop. Simply combine the ingredients in a heavy-based flameproof casserole dish and pour in 2 cups (500 ml) water. Cover and simmer over low heat for about 1 hour or until the chicken is cooked and the sauce has reduced by half. Check it every now and then and give it a good stir.

UNITS PER SERVE					
BREADS, CEREALS, LEGUMES, STARCHY VEGETABLES	DAIRY	LEAN MEAT, FISH, POULTRY, EGGS, TOFU	LOW-CARB VEGETABLES	MODERATE-CARB VEGETABLES	HEALTHY FATS
0	0	1.5	3	1	2

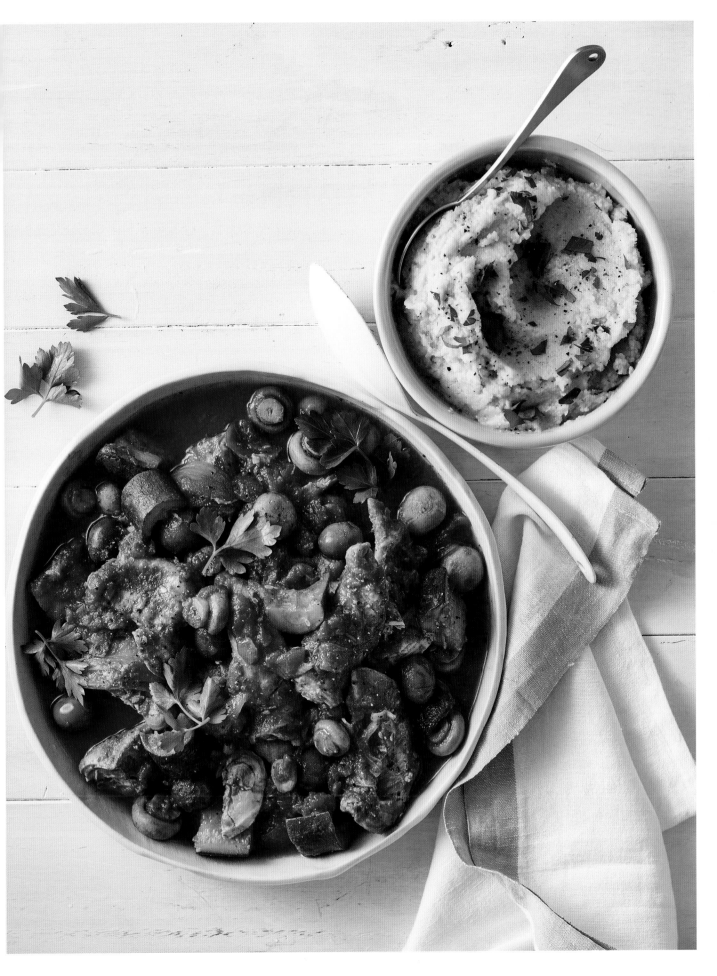

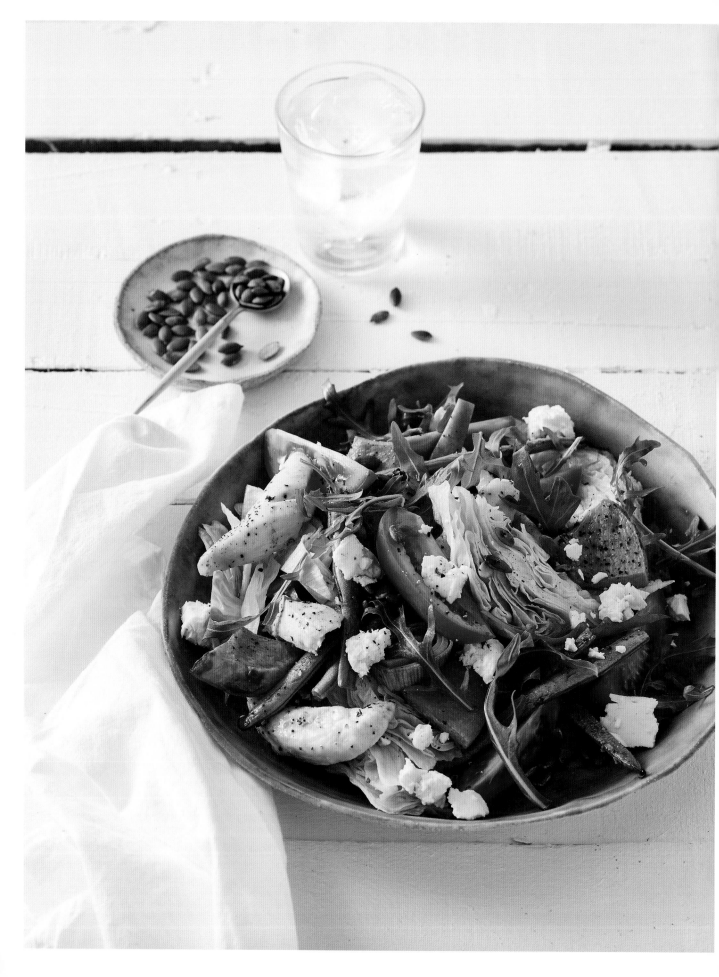

Warm roast chicken *and* pumpkin salad

GRAMS CARB
11
PER SERVE

🍴 Serves 4   🕐 Preparation: 25 minutes, plus 5 minutes standing time
🔥 Cooking: 30 minutes   👨‍🍳 Difficulty: Low

600 g lean chicken tenderloins,
   halved diagonally
150 g peeled, seeded pumpkin,
   cut into 2 cm pieces
2 leeks, white part only, sliced
2 tablespoons olive oil
2 tablespoons no-oil Italian dressing
200 g baby green beans, trimmed
80 g pumpkin seeds (pepitas)
150 g baby rocket leaves
150 g iceberg lettuce, thickly shredded
6 roma tomatoes, quartered
   lengthways
80 g Greek feta, crumbled

Preheat the oven to 200°C (180°C fan-forced).

Place the chicken, pumpkin, leek, oil and dressing in a large roasting tin and toss to combine and coat. Season with freshly ground black pepper. Roast for 20 minutes, then add the beans and pumpkin seeds and roast for a further 10 minutes or until cooked and golden.

Remove the tin from the oven and stand for 5 minutes. Add the rocket, lettuce and tomato and gently toss to combine. Sprinkle with the feta and serve.

UNITS PER SERVE

BREADS, CEREALS, LEGUMES, STARCHY VEGETABLES	DAIRY	LEAN MEAT, FISH, POULTRY, EGGS, TOFU	LOW-CARB VEGETABLES	MODERATE-CARB VEGETABLES	HEALTHY FATS
0	1	1.5	2	1	2

Chermoula chicken *with* asparagus

GRAMS CARB 12 PER SERVE

🍴 Serves 4   🕐 Preparation: 20 minutes
🍳 Cooking: 15 minutes   ⑩ Difficulty: Low

600 g lean chicken tenderloins,
  halved diagonally
2 tablespoons Moroccan seasoning
Finely grated zest and juice of 1 lemon
2 tablespoons extra virgin olive oil
2 spring onions, sliced
3 bunches asparagus, trimmed
500 g mixed baby tomatoes, halved
2 tablespoons flat-leaf parsley leaves
2 tablespoons coriander leaves
500 g fresh cauliflower rice (see note)

Place the chicken, seasoning, lemon zest and juice, oil, spring onion, asparagus and tomato in a bowl. Season with freshly ground black pepper and toss well to combine and coat. Spread out evenly on a large non-stick baking tray.

Preheat the oven grill to high. Cook the chicken mixture under the grill, turning occasionally, for 10–12 minutes or until cooked and golden. Remove and sprinkle with the parsley and coriander.

Meanwhile, heat the cauliflower rice according to the packet instructions.

Divide the cauliflower rice among plates, top with the chicken mixture and serve.

Note: You can find fresh cauliflower rice in the fresh produce section at your local supermarket. If unavailable, use the frozen variety instead.

UNITS PER SERVE

BREADS, CEREALS, LEGUMES, STARCHY VEGETABLES	DAIRY	LEAN MEAT, FISH, POULTRY, EGGS, TOFU	LOW-CARB VEGETABLES	MODERATE-CARB VEGETABLES	HEALTHY FATS
0	0	1.5	2	1	2

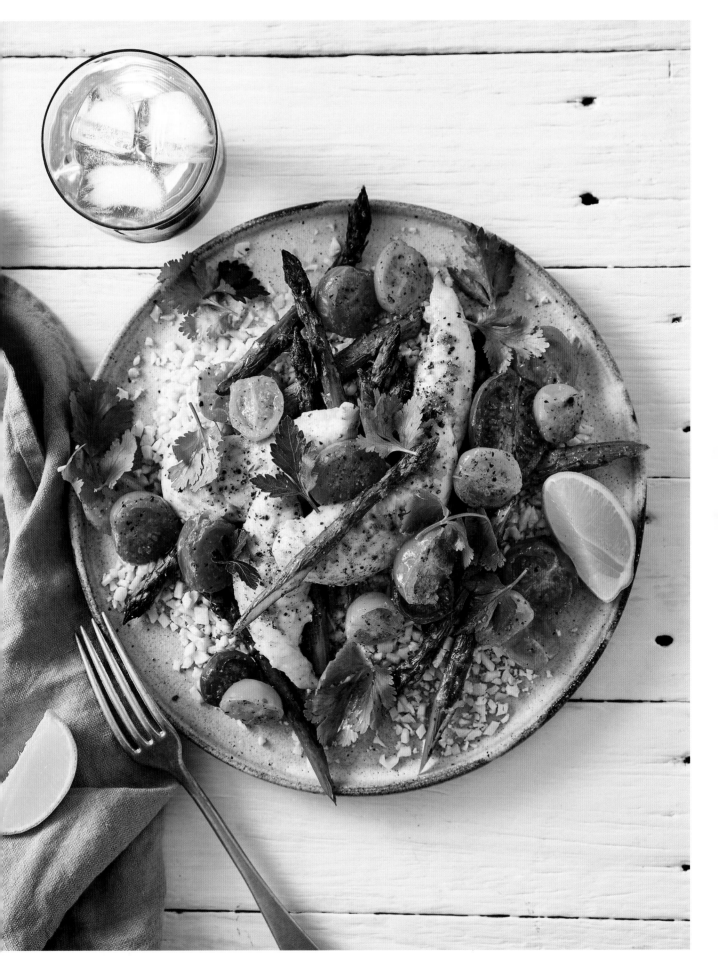

Chicken *and* fennel braise

GRAMS CARB
7
PER SERVE

🍴 Serves 4   🕐 Preparation: 20 minutes, plus 5 minutes resting time
🍳 Cooking: 25 minutes   👨‍🍳 Difficulty: Low

4 x 150 g lean chicken breast fillets

4 small zucchini, thickly sliced
  diagonally

2 tablespoons olive oil

2 cloves garlic, crushed

1 leek, white part only, sliced

1 tablespoon Tuscan dried herb blend

2 bulbs baby fennel, cored and
  thinly sliced

1 cup (250 ml) salt-reduced
  chicken stock

2 tablespoons dill fronds

Preheat a large chargrill pan over medium–high heat. Season the chicken with freshly ground black pepper, then add to the pan and cook, turning occasionally, for 10–12 minutes or until cooked and golden. Transfer to a board, cover loosely with foil and rest for 5 minutes before thickly slicing.

Return the pan to the heat. Chargrill the zucchini, turning occasionally, for 3–5 minutes or until just tender and golden.

Meanwhile, heat the oil in a large deep non-stick frying pan over high heat. Add the garlic, leek, herb blend and fennel and cook, tossing, for 2 minutes. Reduce the heat to low and pour in the stock. Stir well, then cover and simmer very gently, stirring occasionally, for 15 minutes or until the fennel is very tender and the stock has reduced by half.

Divide the fennel mixture, chicken and zucchini among shallow bowls. Sprinkle with the dill and serve.

UNITS PER SERVE

BREADS, CEREALS, LEGUMES, STARCHY VEGETABLES	DAIRY	LEAN MEAT, FISH, POULTRY, EGGS, TOFU	LOW-CARB VEGETABLES	MODERATE-CARB VEGETABLES	HEALTHY FATS
0	0	1.5	2	1	2

Warm chicken *and* bean sprout salad

GRAMS CARB
8
PER SERVE

🍴 Serves 4   🕐 Preparation: 30 minutes
🍲 Cooking: 10 minutes   👨‍🍳 Difficulty: Medium

600 g lean chicken breast fillet,
   roughly chopped
2 teaspoons green curry paste
500 g fresh cauliflower rice (see note)

BEAN SPROUT SALAD
1 tablespoon extra virgin olive oil
2 tablespoons salt-reduced soy sauce
300 g Chinese cabbage (wombok),
   finely shredded
300 g bean sprouts
2 Lebanese cucumbers, halved
   lengthways and thinly sliced
80 g toasted unsalted cashews,
   chopped
4 spring onions, thinly sliced
   into rounds

To make the bean sprout salad, whisk together the oil and soy sauce in a large bowl. Add the remaining ingredients and toss well to combine and coat. Set aside at room temperature.

Process the chicken in a food processor until finely minced.

Heat 1 teaspoon curry paste in a large non-stick wok over high heat. Add the cauliflower rice and stir-fry for 2 minutes or until heated through. Transfer to the bean sprout salad and toss to combine.

Heat the remaining paste in the wok over high heat. Add the chicken and stir-fry, breaking up any lumps with the back of a spoon, for 5–6 minutes or until cooked and light golden. Season with freshly ground black pepper. Transfer to the bean sprout salad and toss through.

Divide the salad among bowls and serve warm.

Note: You can find fresh cauliflower rice in the fresh produce section at your local supermarket. If unavailable, use the frozen variety instead.

UNITS PER SERVE

BREADS, CEREALS, LEGUMES, STARCHY VEGETABLES	DAIRY	LEAN MEAT, FISH, POULTRY, EGGS, TOFU	LOW-CARB VEGETABLES	MODERATE-CARB VEGETABLES	HEALTHY FATS
0	0	1.5	2	1	4

Ginger chicken *and* bok choy bake

GRAMS CARB
7
PER SERVE

🍴 Serves 4   🕐 Preparation: 25 minutes
〰️ Cooking: 25 minutes   👨‍🍳 Difficulty: Low

2 bunches (6 pieces) baby bok choy, halved lengthways
1 red capsicum, seeded and sliced
2 cloves garlic, sliced
7 cm piece ginger, finely grated
¼ cup (60 ml) salt-reduced soy sauce
½ cup (125 ml) salt-reduced chicken stock
600 g lean chicken tenderloins
500 g fresh zucchini noodles (see note)
2 spring onions, thinly sliced
2 tablespoons toasted sesame seeds

Preheat the oven to 200°C (180°C fan-forced).

Place the bok choy, capsicum, garlic, ginger, soy sauce, stock and chicken in a roasting tin and toss well to combine and coat. Bake, tossing occasionally, for 20–25 minutes or until cooked and golden.

Meanwhile, heat the zucchini noodles according to the packet instructions.

Divide the zucchini noodles among large bowls and top with the chicken mixture. Sprinkle with the spring onion and sesame seeds and serve.

Note: You'll find fresh zucchini noodles in the fresh produce section at the supermarket. If unavailable, you can simply cut 4 zucchini into thin matchsticks and lightly steam.

UNITS PER SERVE

BREADS, CEREALS, LEGUMES, STARCHY VEGETABLES	DAIRY	LEAN MEAT, FISH, POULTRY, EGGS, TOFU	LOW-CARB VEGETABLES	MODERATE-CARB VEGETABLES	HEALTHY FATS
0	0	1.5	2	2	2

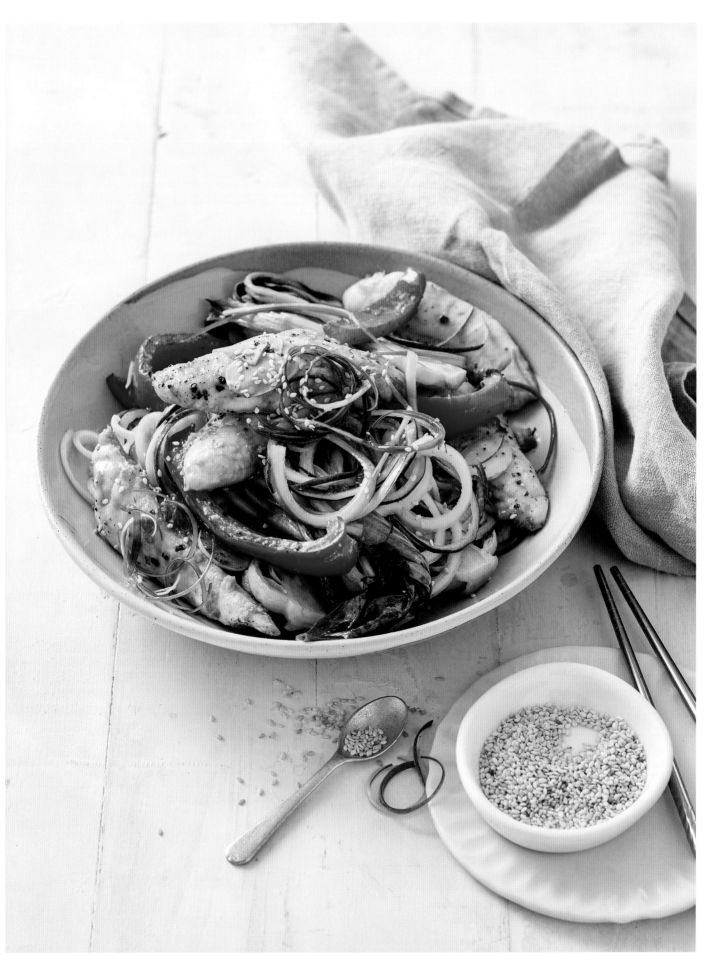

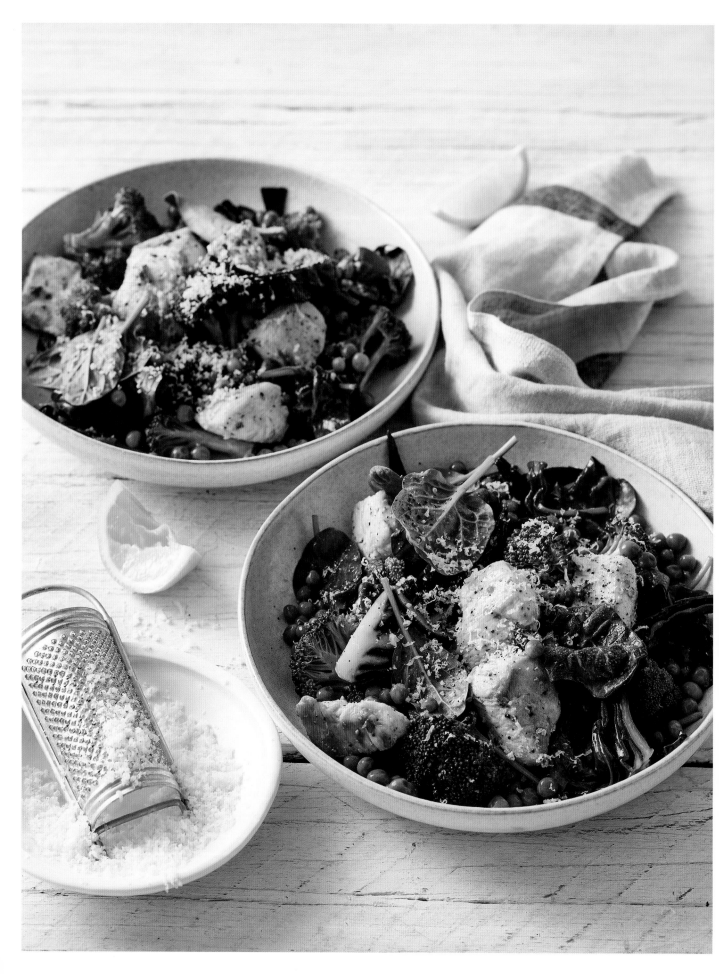

One-pan lemony chicken *and* vegetables

GRAMS CARB
6
PER SERVE

🍴 Serves 4   🕐 Preparation: 25 minutes, plus 5 minutes resting time
🍲 Cooking: 25 minutes   👨‍🍳 Difficulty: Low

600 g lean chicken breast fillets,
   cut into 2 cm pieces
Finely grated zest and juice of
   1 large lemon
2 cloves garlic, crushed
¼ cup (60 ml) olive oil
600 g broccoli florets
2⅔ cups (300 g) shredded red
   cabbage
½ cup (125 ml) salt-reduced chicken
   stock
1 cup frozen baby peas
300 g baby spinach leaves
80 g parmesan, finely grated

Combine the chicken, lemon zest, garlic and 1 tablespoon oil in a large bowl. Season with freshly ground black pepper.

Heat a large deep non-stick frying pan over high heat, add the chicken in three batches and cook for 3 minutes each. Transfer to a clean bowl.

Heat the remaining oil in the pan and return to high heat. Add the broccoli and cabbage and cook, tossing, for 3 minutes or until starting to soften. Return all the chicken to the pan.

Pour in the stock and stir well, then cover and cook, tossing occasionally, for 10 minutes. Remove the pan from the heat and stir through the peas and lemon juice. Rest the baby spinach on top and stand, covered and untouched, for 5 minutes or until the spinach has wilted. Sprinkle with the parmesan and serve.

UNITS PER SERVE

BREADS, CEREALS, LEGUMES, STARCHY VEGETABLES	DAIRY	LEAN MEAT, FISH, POULTRY, EGGS, TOFU	LOW-CARB VEGETABLES	MODERATE-CARB VEGETABLES	HEALTHY FATS
0	1	1.5	2	1	3

Barbecued chicken *and* limes with spiced carrots

GRAMS CARB
8
PER SERVE

🍴 Serves 4   🕐 Preparation: 20 minutes
〰 Cooking: 15 minutes   👨‍🍳 Difficulty: Low

600 g lean chicken breast fillets,
   thickly sliced crossways
4 bunches broccolini, trimmed
4 limes, halved

SPICED CARROTS
2 tablespoons olive oil margarine
2 teaspoons ground cumin
2 tablespoons chopped coriander
4 carrots, cut into thick matchsticks

To make the spiced carrots, combine the margarine, cumin and coriander in a large bowl and season with freshly ground black pepper. Steam the carrot sticks over boiling water for 10–12 minutes or until just tender. Drain, then add to the bowl. Toss well to combine and coat, then cover and set aside.

Meanwhile, preheat a barbecue chargrill plate to high.

Season the chicken with freshly ground black pepper. Add the chicken and broccolini to the barbecue and chargrill, turning occasionally, for 10–12 minutes or until cooked and golden. Add the lime halves, cut side down, for the last 3 minutes of cooking.

Divide the spiced carrots, broccolini, chicken and limes among plates and serve.

UNITS PER SERVE					
BREADS, CEREALS, LEGUMES, STARCHY VEGETABLES	DAIRY	LEAN MEAT, FISH, POULTRY, EGGS, TOFU	LOW-CARB VEGETABLES	MODERATE-CARB VEGETABLES	HEALTHY FATS
0	0	1.5	2	1	2

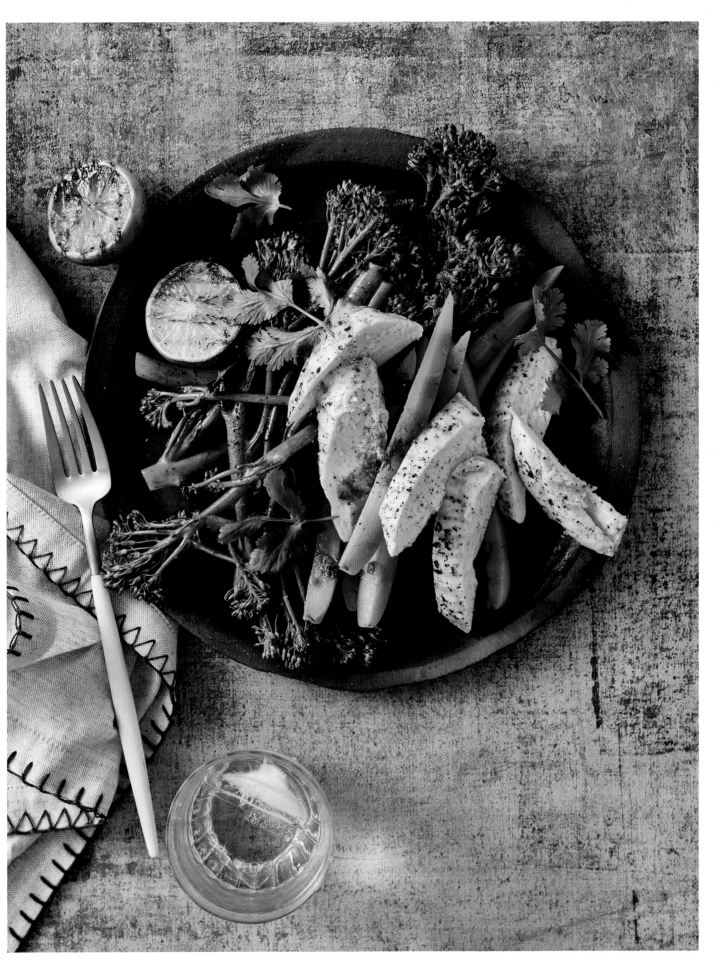

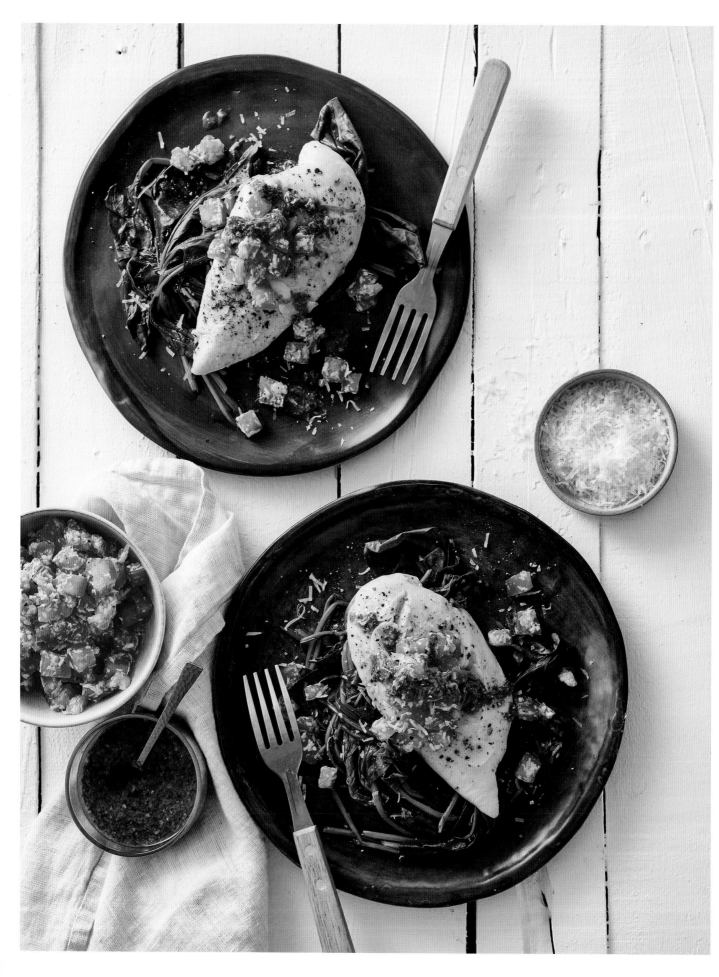

Steam-roasted chicken *with* fresh tomato pesto

GRAMS CARB
7
PER SERVE

🍴 Serves 4 🕐 Preparation: 25 minutes, plus 5 minutes resting time
🥘 Cooking: 15 minutes 🎩 Difficulty: Low

4 x 150 g lean chicken breast
  fillets, scored
2 bunches English spinach,
  leaves picked
4 cloves garlic, sliced
½ cup (125 ml) salt-reduced
  chicken stock

FRESH TOMATO PESTO
1 tablespoon extra virgin olive oil
6 tomatoes, finely chopped
2 tablespoons basil pesto
80 g parmesan, finely grated

Preheat the oven to 200°C (180°C fan-forced).

To make the fresh tomato pesto, combine the oil, tomato, half the basil pesto and half the parmesan in a bowl and season with freshly ground black pepper. Set aside at room temperature, stirring occasionally, until ready to serve.

Season the chicken with freshly ground black pepper. Add the spinach to a large roasting tin and place the chicken on top. Fill the scored sections of the chicken with the garlic slices, then pour the stock into the base of the pan. Cover tightly with baking paper, then a double piece of foil, and roast for 15 minutes or until just cooked. Remove from the oven and stand, covered, for 5 minutes.

Divide the spinach and chicken among plates and spoon over any pan juices. Finish with dollops of the fresh tomato pesto, a drizzle of the remaining basil pesto and a sprinkle of the parmesan, and serve.

UNITS PER SERVE					
BREADS, CEREALS, LEGUMES, STARCHY VEGETABLES	DAIRY	LEAN MEAT, FISH, POULTRY, EGGS, TOFU	LOW-CARB VEGETABLES	MODERATE-CARB VEGETABLES	HEALTHY FATS
0	1	1.5	2	0	3

Roasted meatballs
with tomato olive sauce

GRAMS CARB
(15)
PER SERVE

🍴 Serves 4 🕐 Preparation: 30 minutes
🎯 Cooking: 40 minutes 🍳 Difficulty: Medium

700 g passata with basil
4 zucchini, chopped
1 red onion, finely chopped
1 cup (160 g) pitted small kalamata
   olives
600 g lean chicken breast fillet,
   roughly chopped
2 cloves garlic, crushed
1 teaspoon dried mixed herbs
100 g mozzarella, grated
100 g baby rocket leaves
Lemon wedges, to serve

Preheat the oven to 200°C (180°C fan-forced).

Combine the passata, zucchini, onion and olives in a large roasting tin and roast, covered, for 15 minutes.

Meanwhile, process the chicken, garlic and dried herbs in a food processor until finely minced. Using slightly damp hands, roll the mixture into 12 even meatballs.

Add the meatballs to the tin and roast, uncovered, for 20 minutes or until cooked. Sprinkle the mozzarella over the top and roast for a further 5 minutes or until the cheese has melted. Serve with the rocket leaves and the lemon wedges on the side.

UNITS PER SERVE

BREADS, CEREALS, LEGUMES, STARCHY VEGETABLES	DAIRY	LEAN MEAT, FISH, POULTRY, EGGS, TOFU	LOW-CARB VEGETABLES	MODERATE-CARB VEGETABLES	HEALTHY FATS
0	1	1.5	3	<0.5	2

Bocconcini stuffed chicken tray bake

GRAMS CARB
10
PER SERVE

🍴 **Serves 4**   🕐 **Preparation: 30 minutes, plus 5 minutes standing time**
🍳 **Cooking: 25 minutes**   👨‍🍳 **Difficulty: Medium**

300 g brussels sprouts, trimmed
    and halved
300 g red capsicum, seeded and
    thickly sliced
4 zucchini, sliced into rounds
1 bunch broccolini, trimmed
2 tablespoons olive oil
2 tablespoons salt-reduced garlic and
    herb seasoning
4 x 150 g lean chicken breast fillets
100 g baby bocconcini, sliced
2 tablespoons basil pesto

Preheat the oven to 200°C (180°C fan-forced) and line a large baking tray with baking paper.

Place the brussels sprouts, capsicum, zucchini, broccolini, 1½ tablespoons oil and 1½ tablespoons garlic and herb seasoning on the prepared tray. Toss together to combine and coat evenly, then spread out in a single layer.

Cut each chicken breast through the centre to butterfly and open out flat. Place the bocconcini on one half and season with freshly ground black pepper, then fold the other half over to cover and secure with toothpicks. Nestle among the vegetables on the tray. Drizzle the remaining oil over the chicken, then sprinkle with the remaining seasoning.

Bake for 20–25 minutes or until cooked and golden. Remove from the oven and stand for 5 minutes, then remove and discard the toothpicks. Drizzle over the pesto, then take the tray straight to the table and serve.

UNITS PER SERVE

BREADS, CEREALS, LEGUMES, STARCHY VEGETABLES	DAIRY	LEAN MEAT, FISH, POULTRY, EGGS, TOFU	LOW-CARB VEGETABLES	MODERATE-CARB VEGETABLES	HEALTHY FATS
0	1	1.5	2	1	4

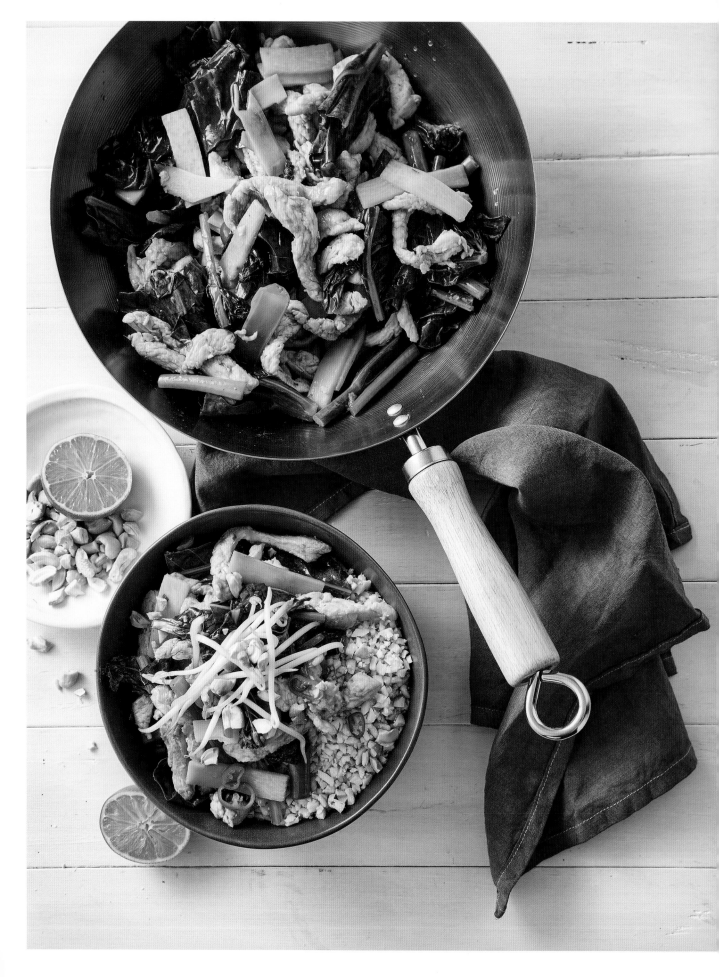

Ginger turkey stir-fry

GRAMS CARB
9
PER SERVE

🍴 Serves 4 🕐 Preparation: 25 minutes
♨ Cooking: 15 minutes 👨‍🍳 Difficulty: Low

1 teaspoon sesame oil
600 g lean turkey breast fillet,
　thinly sliced
5 cm piece ginger, cut into
　thin matchsticks
2 bunches Chinese broccoli, trimmed
　and cut into 4 cm lengths
2 tablespoons salt-reduced soy sauce
225 g tin sliced bamboo shoots,
　drained
2 cups (180 g) bean sprouts
2 long green chillies, thinly sliced
250 g fresh cauliflower rice (see note)
80 g unsalted toasted cashews,
　chopped
Lime wedges, to serve (optional)

Combine the oil, turkey and ginger in a bowl and season with
freshly ground black pepper.

Heat a large non-stick wok over high heat. Add the turkey in three
batches and stir-fry for 3–4 minutes each or until just cooked and
golden. Transfer to a clean bowl.

Add the broccoli, soy sauce and bamboo shoots to the wok and
stir-fry for 2–3 minutes or until just wilted. Return the turkey to the
wok and toss to combine. Remove the wok from the heat and toss
through the bean sprouts and chilli.

Meanwhile, heat the cauliflower rice according to the packet
instructions.

Divide the cauliflower rice and turkey stir-fry among bowls, sprinkle
with the cashews and serve with the lime wedges, if desired.

Note: You can find fresh cauliflower rice in the fresh produce
section at your local supermarket. If unavailable, use the frozen
variety instead.

UNITS PER SERVE

BREADS, CEREALS, LEGUMES, STARCHY VEGETABLES	DAIRY	LEAN MEAT, FISH, POULTRY, EGGS, TOFU	LOW-CARB VEGETABLES	MODERATE-CARB VEGETABLES	HEALTHY FATS
0	0	1.5	2	1	2

Roast Thai pork *and* broccoli

GRAMS CARB
9
PER SERVE

🍴 Serves 4   🕐 Preparation: 25 minutes, plus 5 minutes resting time
🍲 Cooking: 30 minutes   🎩 Difficulty: Low

600 g broccoli florets
4 small zucchini, sliced
2 tablespoons fresh Thai herb paste
2 tablespoons salt-reduced soy sauce
1 tablespoon olive oil
600 g lean pork fillet
½ cup coriander leaves
80 g toasted unsalted cashews, chopped
Lime wedges, to serve

Preheat the oven to 200°C (180°C fan-forced) and line a large baking tray with baking paper.

Place the broccoli and zucchini on the prepared tray in a single layer and season with freshly ground black pepper.

Combine the herb paste, soy sauce and oil in a bowl, add the pork fillet and turn to coat evenly on all sides. Transfer the mixture to the tray, placing the pork fillet on top of the vegetables.

Roast for 25–30 minutes or until cooked and golden. Remove the tray from the oven, cover loosely with foil and rest for 5 minutes before thickly slicing the pork.

Divide the pork, vegetables and any pan juices among plates. Sprinkle with the coriander leaves and cashews and serve with the lime wedges.

UNITS PER SERVE

BREADS, CEREALS, LEGUMES, STARCHY VEGETABLES	DAIRY	LEAN MEAT, FISH, POULTRY, EGGS, TOFU	LOW-CARB VEGETABLES	MODERATE-CARB VEGETABLES	HEALTHY FATS
0	0	1.5	2	0	3

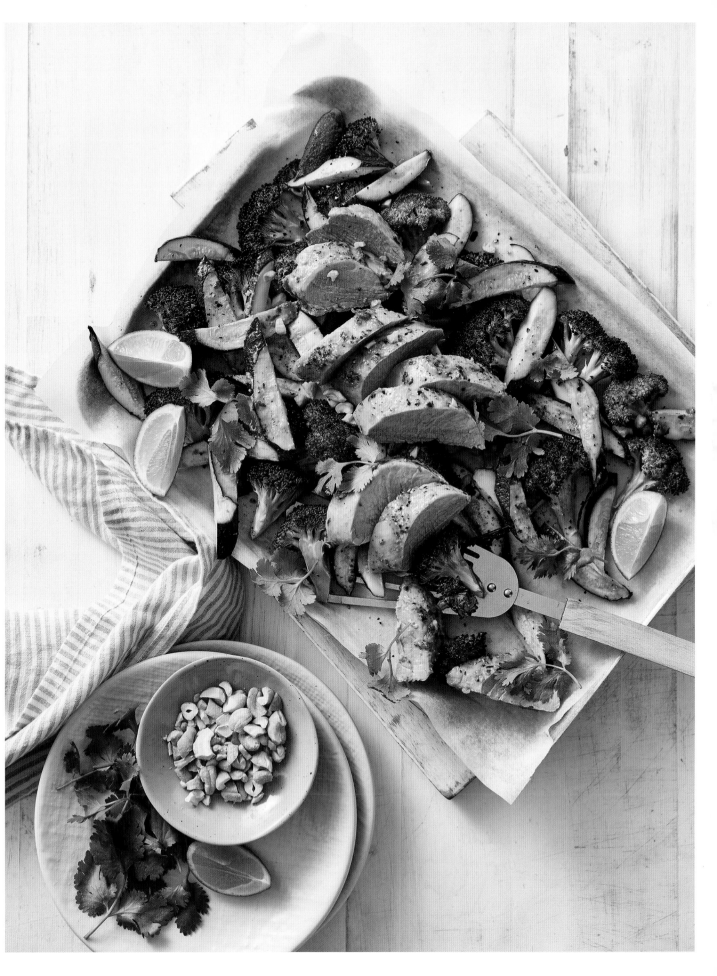

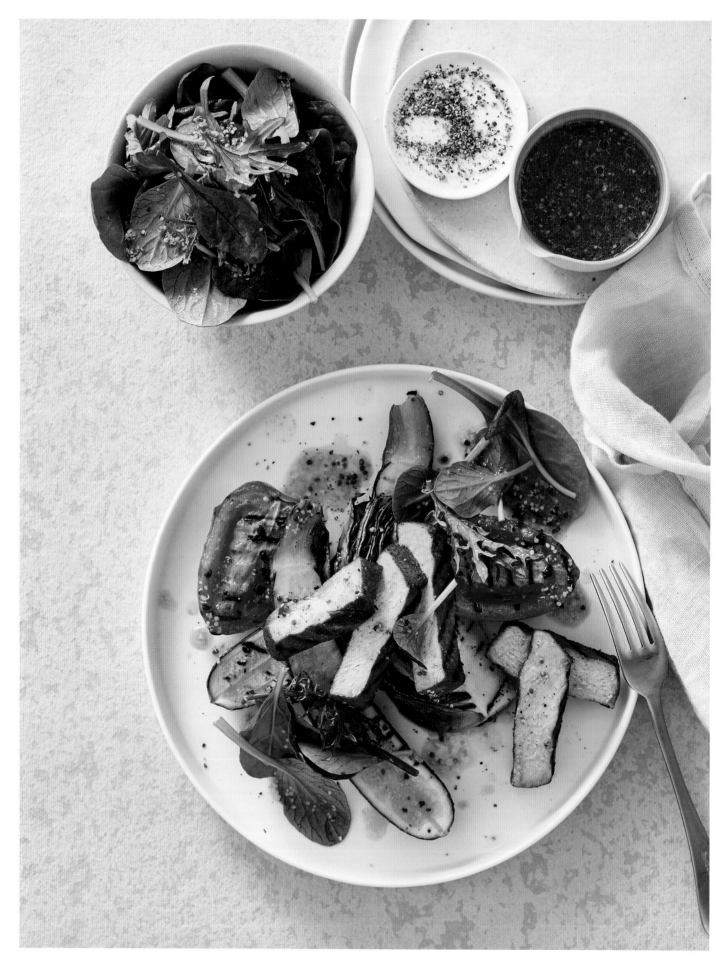

Smoky pork *and* barbecued cabbage *with* mustard dressing

🍴 Serves 4   🕐 Preparation: 20 minutes
〰 Cooking: 15 minutes   🎖 Difficulty: Low

4 x 150 g lean pork loin steaks
1 tablespoon smoked paprika
600 g piece small red cabbage,
   cut into 4 equal wedges
4 small zucchini, halved lengthways
4 roma tomatoes, halved horizontally
150 g mixed salad leaves

MUSTARD DRESSING
1 tablespoon wholegrain mustard
2 tablespoons extra virgin olive oil
⅓ cup (80 ml) red wine vinegar

To make the mustard dressing, whisk together all the ingredients in a small jug. Season with freshly ground black pepper.

Preheat a barbecue chargrill plate to high. Season the steaks with freshly ground black pepper and sprinkle evenly with the paprika. Set aside.

Chargrill the cabbage and zucchini for 5 minutes, turning occasionally. Add the steaks and tomato halves and chargrill, turning occasionally, for a further 10 minutes or until cooked and golden.

Divide the salad leaves, pork and vegetables among plates, spoon over the mustard dressing and serve.

UNITS PER SERVE

BREADS, CEREALS, LEGUMES, STARCHY VEGETABLES	DAIRY	LEAN MEAT, FISH, POULTRY, EGGS, TOFU	LOW-CARB VEGETABLES	MODERATE-CARB VEGETABLES	HEALTHY FATS
0	0	1.5	2	1	2

4

SEAFOOD & VEGETARIAN DINNERS

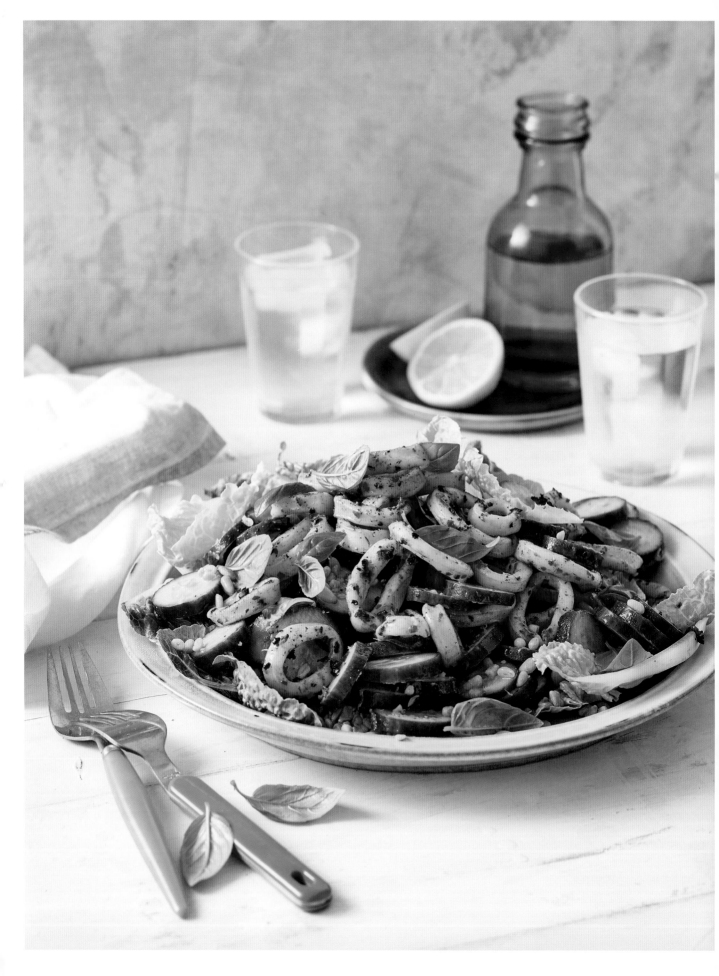

Chilli squid *with* nutty cucumber salad

GRAMS CARB
7
PER SERVE

🍴 Serves 4   🕐 Preparation: 30 minutes
♨ Cooking: 5 minutes   👨‍🍳 Difficulty: Low

600 g cleaned fresh squid hoods,
   sliced into rings
2 long red chillies, finely chopped
1 clove garlic, crushed
1 tablespoon olive oil

NUTTY CUCUMBER SALAD
1 tablespoon extra virgin olive oil
Finely grated zest and juice of
   1 small lemon
6 Lebanese cucumbers, very thinly
   sliced into rounds
½ cup small basil leaves
2 baby cos lettuces, chopped
80 g toasted pine nuts,
   roughly chopped

Combine the squid, chilli, garlic and oil in a bowl and season with freshly ground black pepper. Chill until required.

To make the nutty cucumber salad, place all the ingredients in a large bowl, season with freshly ground black pepper and toss to combine. Divide among serving plates.

Heat a large chargrill pan over high heat. Add the squid and cook, turning constantly, for 2–3 minutes or until just tender. Transfer to the plates with the salad and serve.

UNITS PER SERVE

BREADS, CEREALS, LEGUMES, STARCHY VEGETABLES	DAIRY	LEAN MEAT, FISH, POULTRY, EGGS, TOFU	LOW-CARB VEGETABLES	MODERATE-CARB VEGETABLES	HEALTHY FATS
0	0	1.5	2	0	4

Hoisin barramundi bowls

🍴 Serves 4   🕐 Preparation: 20 minutes
〰 Cooking: 15 minutes   👨‍🍳 Difficulty: Low

600 g skinless, boneless barramundi
   fillets, cut into 4 cm pieces
2 tablespoons hoisin sauce
1 tablespoon soy sauce
1 tablespoon olive oil
Lime wedges, to serve (optional)

WOK-TOSSED VEGGIES
1 tablespoon sunflower oil
1 red onion, cut into thin wedges
300 g snow peas, trimmed
300 g sugar snap peas, trimmed
1 bunch kale, white stalks removed,
   torn
2 cloves garlic, crushed

Preheat the oven grill to high.

Place the barramundi, hoisin, soy sauce and olive oil in a large bowl and toss to coat evenly. Place on a large non-stick baking tray in a single layer and cook under the grill, turning occasionally, for 10–12 minutes or until cooked and golden.

Meanwhile, for the wok-tossed veggies, heat half the sunflower oil in a large non-stick wok over high heat. Add the onion, snow peas and sugar snaps and stir-fry for 3–4 minutes or until just tender. Transfer to a large bowl. Add the remaining oil to the wok. Once hot, add the kale and garlic and stir-fry for 1–2 minutes or until wilted. Add to the bowl and toss to combine.

Divide the vegetables among bowls, top with the barramundi and serve with the lime wedges, if desired.

UNITS PER SERVE

BREADS, CEREALS, LEGUMES, STARCHY VEGETABLES	DAIRY	LEAN MEAT, FISH, POULTRY, EGGS, TOFU	LOW-CARB VEGETABLES	MODERATE-CARB VEGETABLES	HEALTHY FATS
0	0	1.5	2	1	2

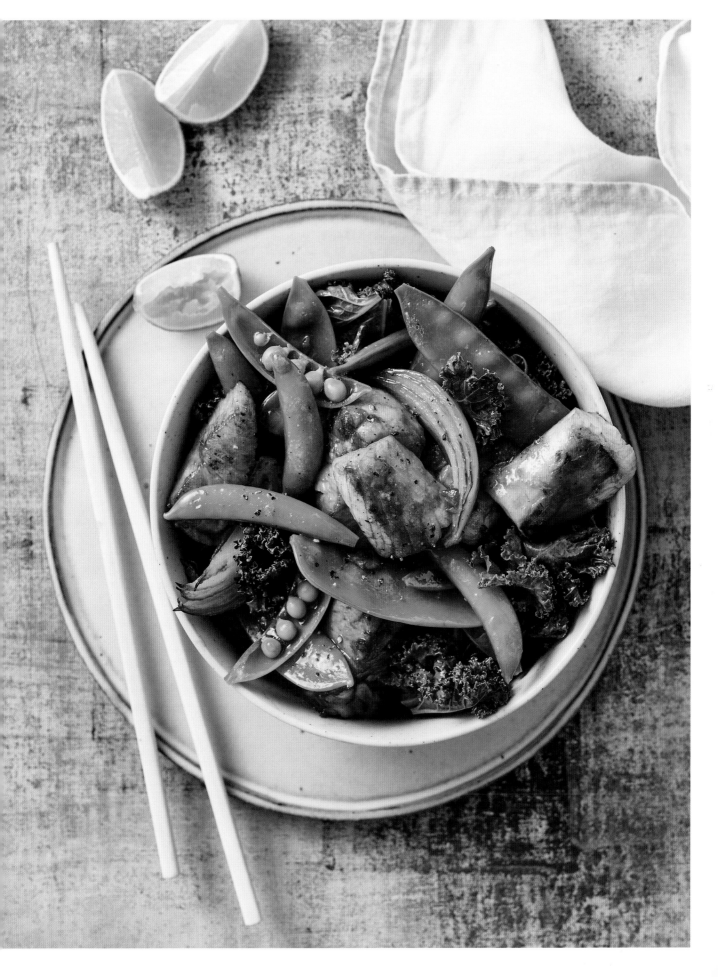

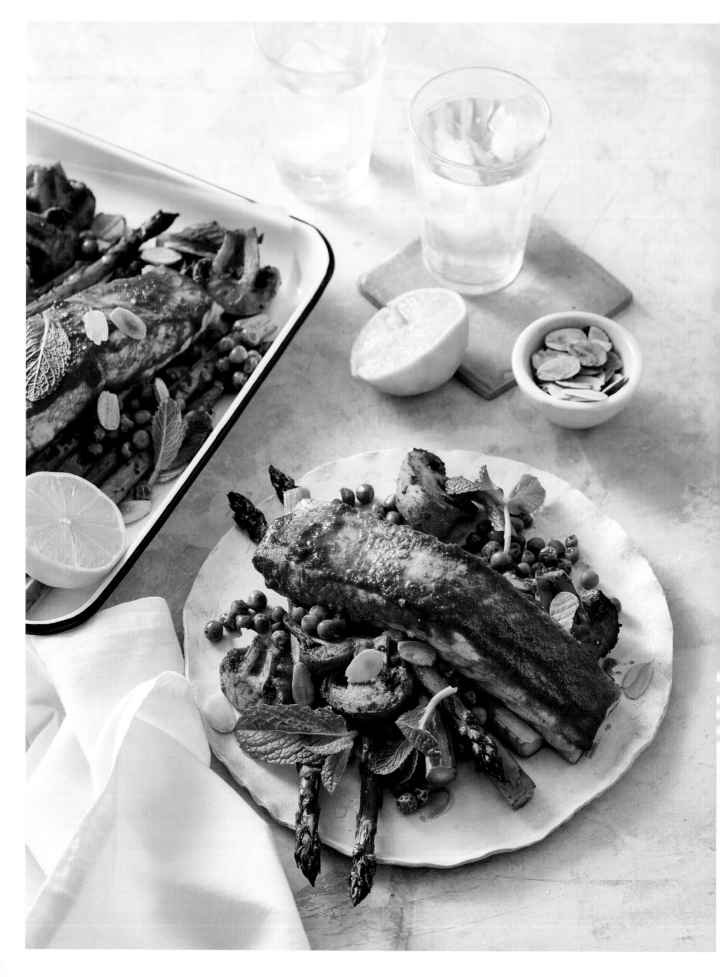

Tandoori salmon tray bake

Serves 4   **Preparation: 25 minutes**
Cooking: 20 minutes   **Difficulty: Low**

2 tablespoons tandoori paste
Finely grated zest and juice of 1 large
    lemon, plus extra wedges to serve
4 x 150 g skinless, boneless
    salmon fillets
3 bunches asparagus, trimmed
600 g cup mushrooms, halved
Olive oil spray, for cooking
1 cup frozen baby peas
40 g flaked almonds
½ cup small mint leaves

Preheat the oven to 200°C (180°C fan-forced) and line a large baking tray with baking paper.

Whisk together the tandoori paste, lemon zest and juice in a large bowl. Add the salmon and toss well to coat. Transfer the salmon to the prepared tray. Place the asparagus and mushrooms in the bowl with the remaining tandoori mixture and toss well to coat. Transfer to the tray, in and around the salmon pieces, then lightly spray everything with the olive oil.

Bake for 10 minutes, then add the peas and almonds and bake for a further 8–10 minutes or until cooked and golden.

Remove the tray from the oven, sprinkle with the mint leaves and serve with the lemon wedges.

UNITS PER SERVE

BREADS, CEREALS, LEGUMES, STARCHY VEGETABLES	DAIRY	LEAN MEAT, FISH, POULTRY, EGGS, TOFU	LOW-CARB VEGETABLES	MODERATE-CARB VEGETABLES	HEALTHY FATS
0	0	1.5	2	1	3

Summer pesto prawns *with* zucchini noodles

GRAMS CARB
8
PER SERVE

🍴 Serves 4   🕐 Preparation: 20 minutes, plus 30 minutes chilling time
🎩 Difficulty: Low

80 g basil pesto
Finely grated zest and juice of
    1 large lemon
600 g cooked peeled, deveined
    medium tiger prawns
600 g mixed baby tomatoes, halved
500 g fresh zucchini noodles
    (see note)
1 bunch baby radishes, very thinly
    sliced into rounds

Combine the pesto, lemon zest and juice, prawns and tomato in a large bowl and season with freshly ground black pepper. Place in the fridge to marinate for 30 minutes, tossing occasionally.

Add the zucchini noodles and radish to the prawn mixture and toss to combine. Divide among bowls and serve.

Note: You'll find fresh zucchini noodles in the fresh produce section at the supermarket. If unavailable, you can simply cut 4 zucchini into thin matchsticks and lightly steam.

UNITS PER SERVE

BREADS, CEREALS, LEGUMES, STARCHY VEGETABLES	DAIRY	LEAN MEAT, FISH, POULTRY, EGGS, TOFU	LOW-CARB VEGETABLES	MODERATE-CARB VEGETABLES	HEALTHY FATS
0	0	1.5	2	1	4

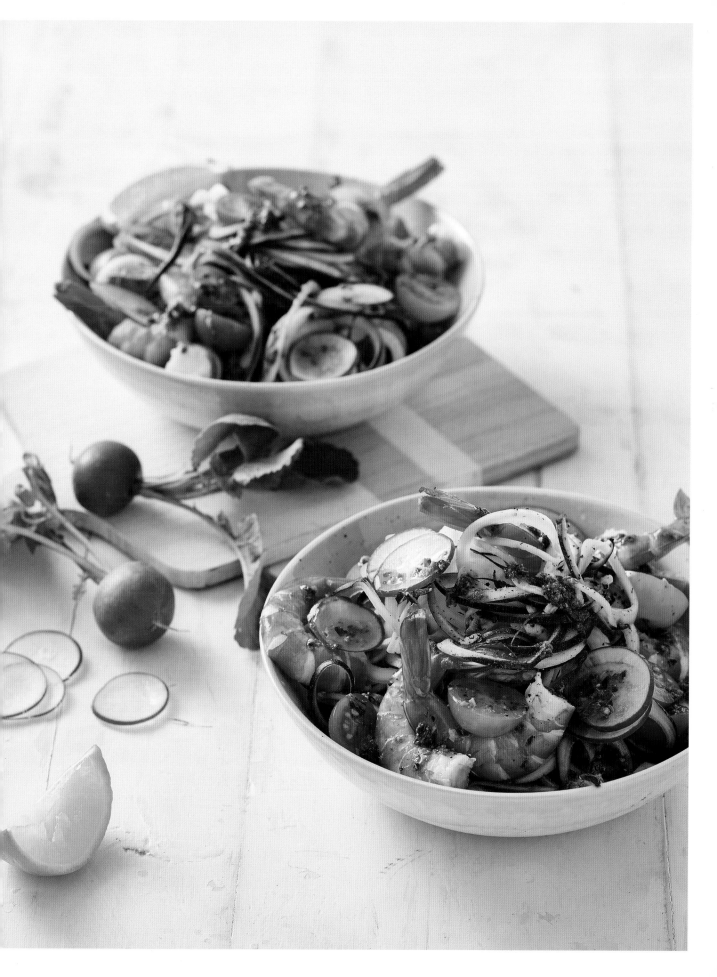

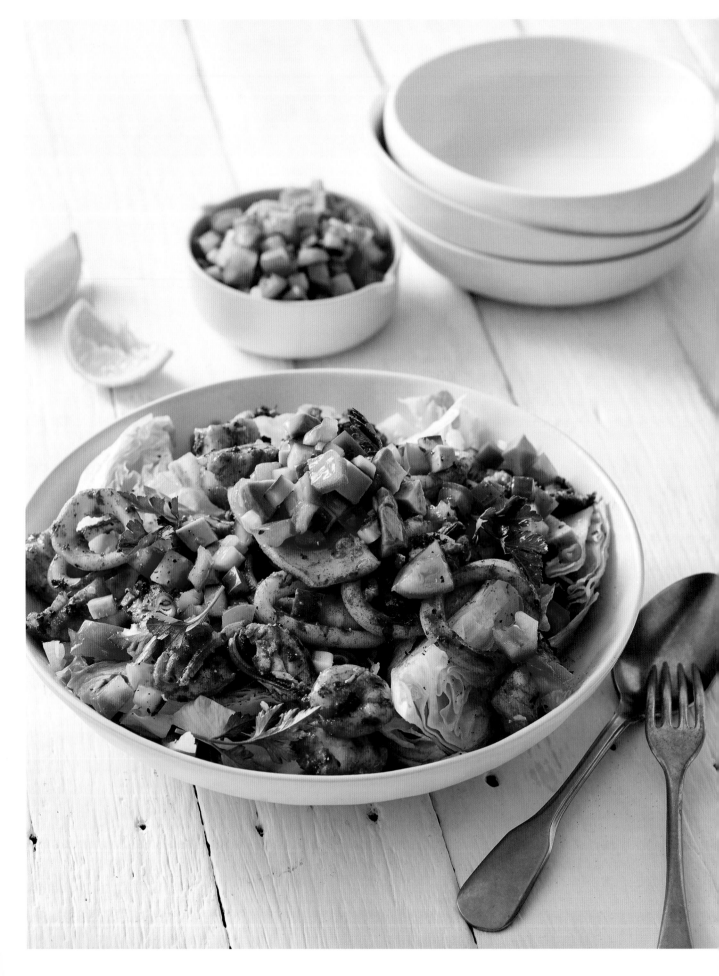

Barbecued marinara *with* fresh salsa dressing

GRAMS CARB
8
PER SERVE

🍴 Serves 4   🕐 Preparation: 30 minutes
🍳 Cooking: 5 minutes   🎩 Difficulty: Low

600 g fresh seafood marinara mix
2 teaspoons smoked paprika
1 small iceberg lettuce, cut into
    wedges
Flat-leaf parsley leaves, to serve

FRESH SALSA DRESSING
⅓ cup (80 ml) oil-free Italian dressing
4 Lebanese cucumbers, finely chopped
2 spring onions, thinly sliced
    into rounds
4 tomatoes, finely chopped
1 green capsicum, seeded and
    finely chopped
160 g avocado, finely chopped

To make the fresh salsa dressing, combine all the ingredients in a bowl and season with freshly ground black pepper. Stand at room temperature until serving.

Preheat a barbecue flat plate to high.

Combine the seafood with the paprika. Add to the barbecue plate and cook, tossing constantly, for 3–5 minutes or until just cooked and golden.

Divide the seafood and iceberg wedges among plates, drizzle over the fresh salsa dressing and serve with the parsley leaves.

UNITS PER SERVE

BREADS, CEREALS, LEGUMES, STARCHY VEGETABLES	DAIRY	LEAN MEAT, FISH, POULTRY, EGGS, TOFU	LOW-CARB VEGETABLES	MODERATE-CARB VEGETABLES	HEALTHY FATS
0	0	1.5	3	1	2

Roast vegetable frittata

GRAMS CARB
9
PER SERVE

🍴 Serves 4   🕐 Preparation: 25 minutes, plus 5 minutes resting time
〰 Cooking: 45 minutes   ⓥ Difficulty: Low

150 g peeled, seeded pumpkin,
cut into 2 cm pieces
600 g broccoli florets
2 bulbs baby fennel, cored and
cut into 2 cm pieces
12 x 55 g eggs, whisked
100 g Greek-style yoghurt
1 bunch chives, finely chopped
220 g fresh ricotta, crumbled
240 g avocado, sliced
Lemon wedges, to serve

Preheat the oven to 200°C (180°C fan-forced) and line a large baking dish (about 30 cm x 22 cm) with baking paper.

Add the pumpkin, broccoli and fennel to the prepared dish and season with freshly ground black pepper. Roast for 20 minutes or until just tender and golden.

Whisk together the eggs, yoghurt and chives, then pour over the roast vegetables. Dot the top with the ricotta, then return to the oven for 20–25 minutes or until golden and the egg is set.

Remove from the oven and rest for 5 minutes. Take to the table and serve with the avocado and lemon wedges.

UNITS PER SERVE

BREADS, CEREALS, LEGUMES, STARCHY VEGETABLES	DAIRY	LEAN MEAT, FISH, POULTRY, EGGS, TOFU	LOW-CARB VEGETABLES	MODERATE-CARB VEGETABLES	HEALTHY FATS
0	1	1.5	2	1	3

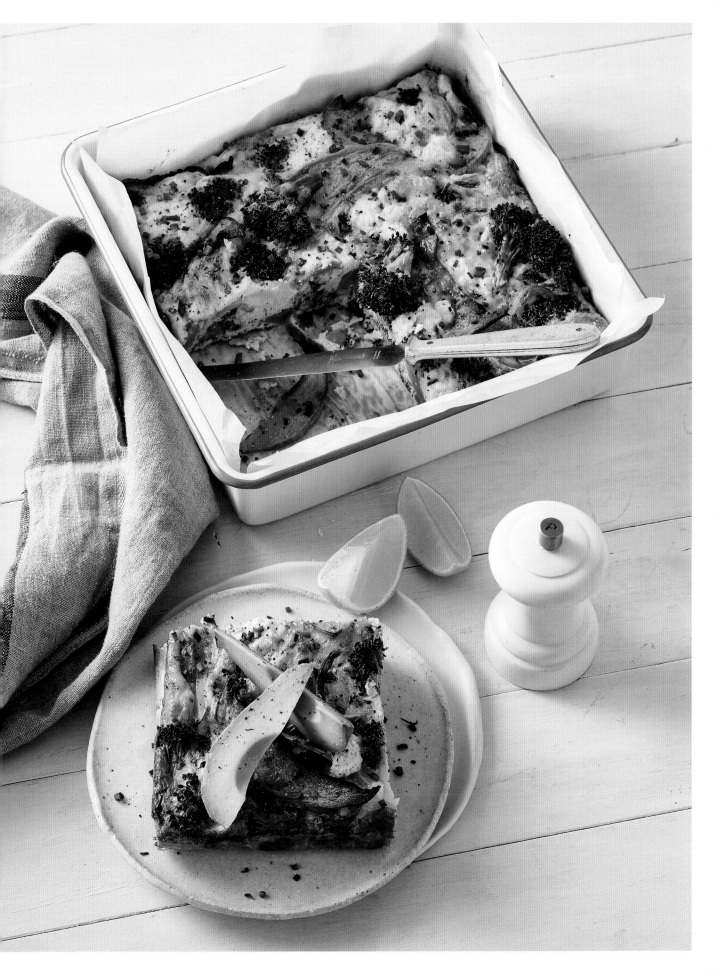

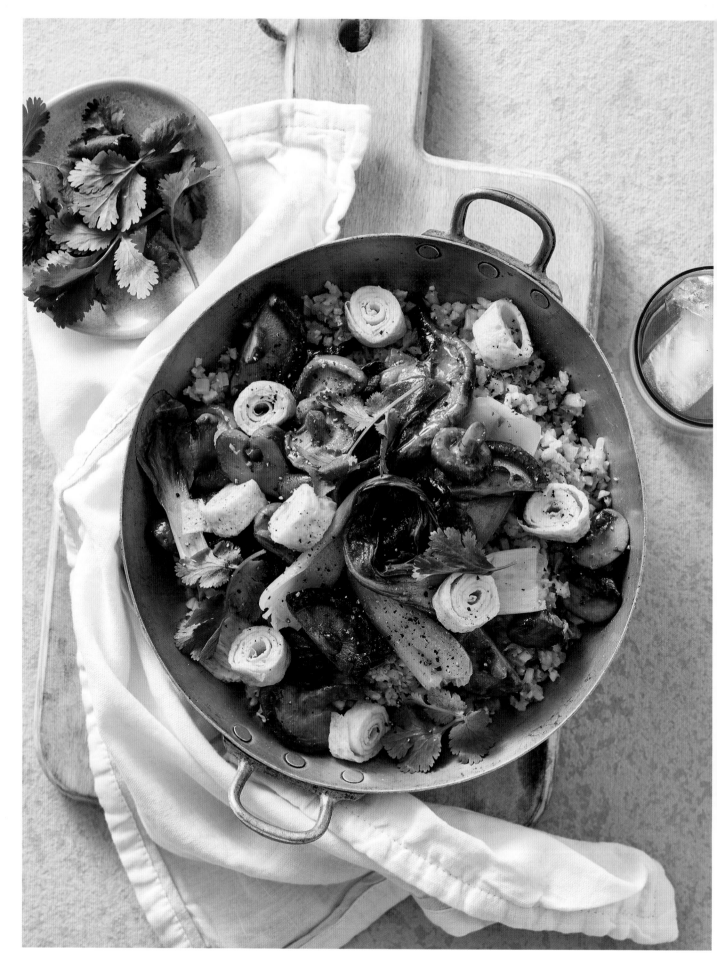

Thai mushroom stir-fry *with* cauliflower omelette rice

GRAMS CARB
10
PER SERVE

🍴 Serves 4   🕐 Preparation: 25 minutes
♨ Cooking: 10 minutes   👨‍🍳 Difficulty: Medium

Olive oil spray, for cooking
12 x 55 g eggs, whisked
500 g fresh cauliflower rice (see note)
2 tablespoons sunflower oil
2 tablespoons fresh Thai herb paste
600 g mixed mushrooms (field,
    portobello, shiitake, button),
    thickly sliced
2 bunches (6 pieces) baby bok choy,
    leaves separated
½ cup coriander leaves

Lightly spray a large non-stick frying pan with the olive oil and heat over high heat. Add one-quarter of the whisked egg and swirl to coat the base of the pan. Cook, untouched, for 2 minutes or until the egg has just set. Carefully slide the omelette onto a board. Repeat with a little more oil spray and the remaining egg to make four omelettes in all. Roll up each omelette to form a log and slice into rounds. Set aside.

Lightly spray the pan with a little more olive oil, add the cauliflower rice and cook, stirring occasionally, for 2 minutes or until heated through. Return the egg strips and toss through, then remove the pan from the heat.

Meanwhile, heat the sunflower oil in a large non-stick wok over high heat. Add the herb paste and mushroom and stir-fry for 1 minute. Add the bok choy and 2 tablespoons water and stir-fry for 2 minutes or until just tender.

Divide the cauliflower omelette rice among bowls and top with the mushroom mixture. Sprinkle with the coriander and serve.

Note: You can purchase fresh cauliflower rice in the fresh produce section at your local supermarket. If unavailable, use the frozen variety instead.

UNITS PER SERVE

BREADS, CEREALS, LEGUMES, STARCHY VEGETABLES	DAIRY	LEAN MEAT, FISH, POULTRY, EGGS, TOFU	LOW-CARB VEGETABLES	MODERATE-CARB VEGETABLES	HEALTHY FATS
0	0	1.5	2	1	4

5

BEEF & LAMB DINNERS

Balsamic marinated beef *with* tomatoes

GRAMS CARB
11
PER SERVE

🍴 Serves 4   🕐 Preparation: 25 minutes, plus 1 hour chilling time
📖 Cooking: 15 minutes   ✋ Difficulty: Low

4 x 150 g lean beef fillet steaks
1 red onion, cut into wedges
600 g cherry tomatoes
8 baby yellow squash, halved
4 baby gem lettuces, quartered
  lengthways
80 g Greek feta, crumbled

BALSAMIC MARINADE
⅓ cup (80 ml) balsamic vinegar
2 tablespoons extra virgin olive oil
2 tablespoons garlic and herb
  seasoning
2 teaspoons Dijon mustard

To make the balsamic marinade, whisk together all the ingredients in a large bowl.

Add the beef, onion, tomatoes and squash to the marinade and toss to combine and coat. Season with freshly ground black pepper. Cover and chill for at least 1 hour or overnight if time permits.

Preheat a large chargrill pan over high heat. Add the onion, tomatoes and squash and chargrill, turning occasionally, for 6–8 minutes or until just tender and golden. Transfer to serving plates.

Chargrill the steaks for 3 minutes each side for medium or until cooked to your liking. Transfer to the plates and add the lettuce. Sprinkle with the feta and serve.

UNITS PER SERVE

BREADS, CEREALS, LEGUMES, STARCHY VEGETABLES	DAIRY	LEAN MEAT, FISH, POULTRY, EGGS, TOFU	LOW-CARB VEGETABLES	MODERATE-CARB VEGETABLES	HEALTHY FATS
0	1	1.5	2	1	2

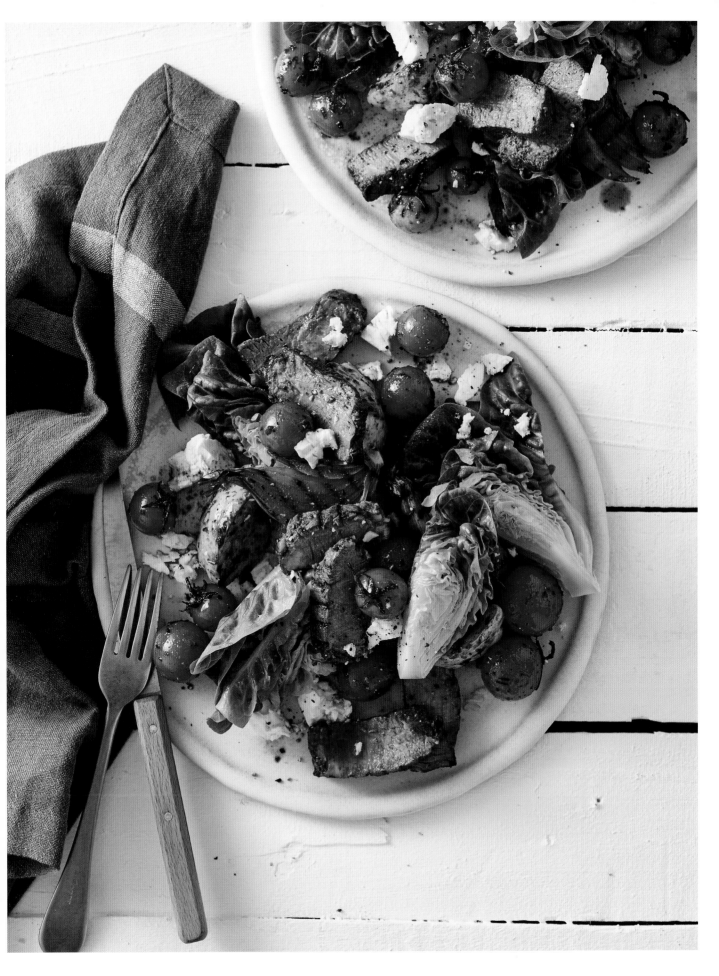

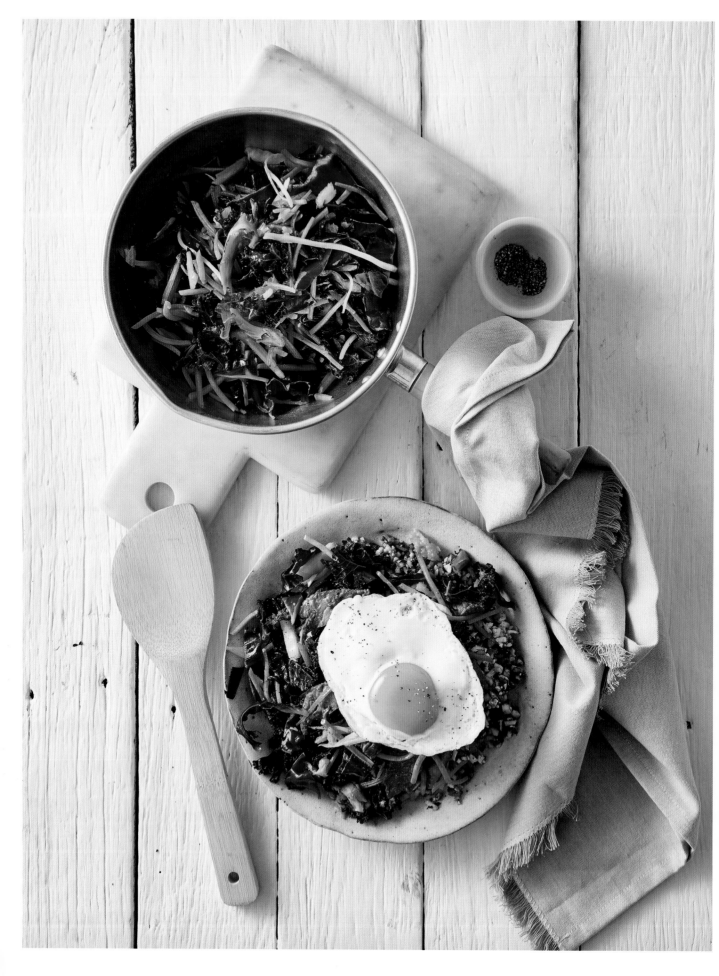

Korean beef

🍴 Serves 4   🕐 Preparation: 20 minutes, plus 30 minutes chilling time
🍳 Cooking: 10 minutes   👨‍🍳 Difficulty: Medium

2 tablespoons salt-reduced soy sauce
2 cloves garlic, crushed
5 cm piece ginger, finely chopped
2 tablespoons sunflower oil
400 g lean rump steak,
     very thinly sliced
4 x 55 g eggs
2 x 375 g fresh shredded
     stir-fry vegetables
2 x 200 g packets fresh cauliflower
     and mushroom 'mince' (see note)

Combine the soy sauce, garlic, ginger and 1 tablespoon oil in a bowl, add the steak and turn to coat well. Cover and marinate in the fridge for at least 30 minutes or overnight if time permits.

Heat 2 teaspoons oil in a large non-stick frying pan over high heat. Add the eggs and cook, untouched, for 3–4 minutes or until the egg whites are set with crisp edges and the yolks are still runny.

Meanwhile, heat a large non-stick wok over high heat. Add the beef in two batches and stir-fry for 2 minutes each or until just cooked and golden. Transfer to a bowl.

Heat the remaining oil in the wok. Add the shredded vegetables and stir-fry for 2 minutes or until just tender. Divide among serving bowls. Add the 'mince' and 2 tablespoons water to the wok and stir-fry for 2 minutes or until just cooked. Transfer to the serving bowls.

Divide the beef among the bowls, top with the fried eggs and serve.

Note: You can find fresh cauliflower and mushroom 'mince' in the fresh produce section at your local supermarket. If unavailable, use the frozen variety of cauliflower rice instead and add 200 g finely chopped field mushrooms.

UNITS PER SERVE

BREADS, CEREALS, LEGUMES, STARCHY VEGETABLES	DAIRY	LEAN MEAT, FISH, POULTRY, EGGS, TOFU	LOW-CARB VEGETABLES	MODERATE-CARB VEGETABLES	HEALTHY FATS
0	0	1.5	2	1	2

Harissa beef skewers *and* zesty herb salad

GRAMS CARB
9
PER SERVE

🍴 Serves 4 🕐 Preparation: 45 minutes
♨ Cooking: 10 minutes 👨‍🍳 Difficulty: Medium

600 g lean beef fillet, cubed
1 red capsicum, seeded and chopped
2 tablespoons harissa spice blend

ZESTY HERB SALAD
1 cup basil leaves
1 cup coriander leaves
½ cup mint leaves
1 cup bean sprouts
2 cups shredded iceberg lettuce
2 Lebanese cucumbers, roughly
  chopped
Finely grated zest and juice of 2 limes
80 g toasted unsalted macadamias,
  chopped

Soak eight bamboo skewers in water for 20 minutes.

Place the beef and capsicum in a bowl, sprinkle over the harissa and toss to combine and coat. Thread the beef and capsicum evenly onto the skewers.

Heat a large chargrill pan over high heat. Add the skewers and cook, turning occasionally, for 8–10 minutes or until just cooked and golden.

Meanwhile, to make the salad, combine all the ingredients in a bowl.

Divide the salad and skewers among plates and serve.

UNITS PER SERVE

BREADS, CEREALS, LEGUMES, STARCHY VEGETABLES	DAIRY	LEAN MEAT, FISH, POULTRY, EGGS, TOFU	LOW-CARB VEGETABLES	MODERATE-CARB VEGETABLES	HEALTHY FATS
0	0	1.5	2	0.5	2

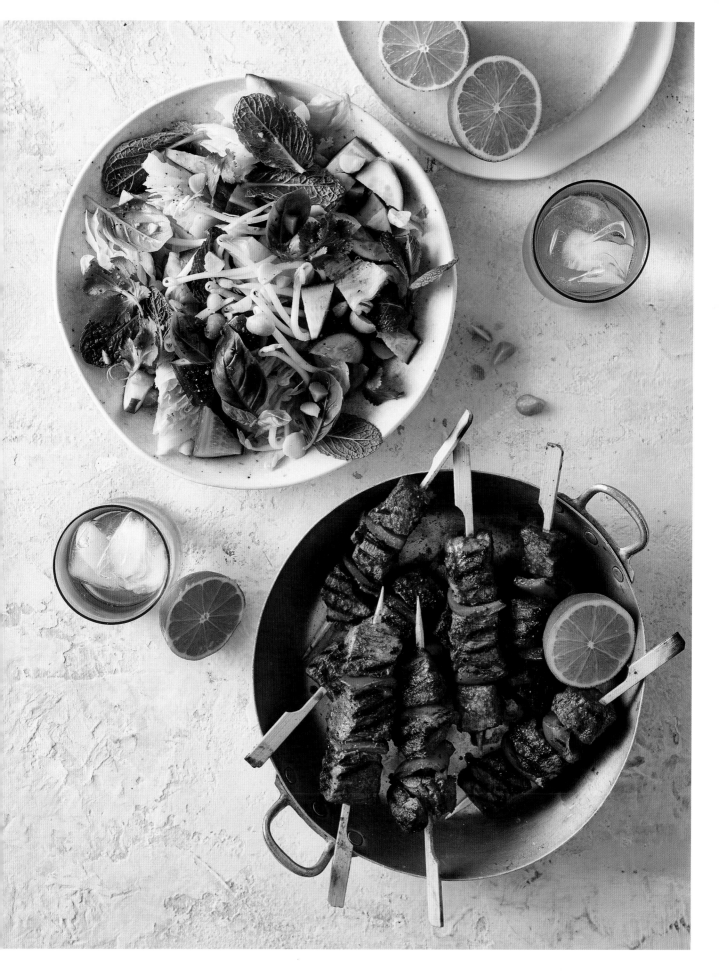

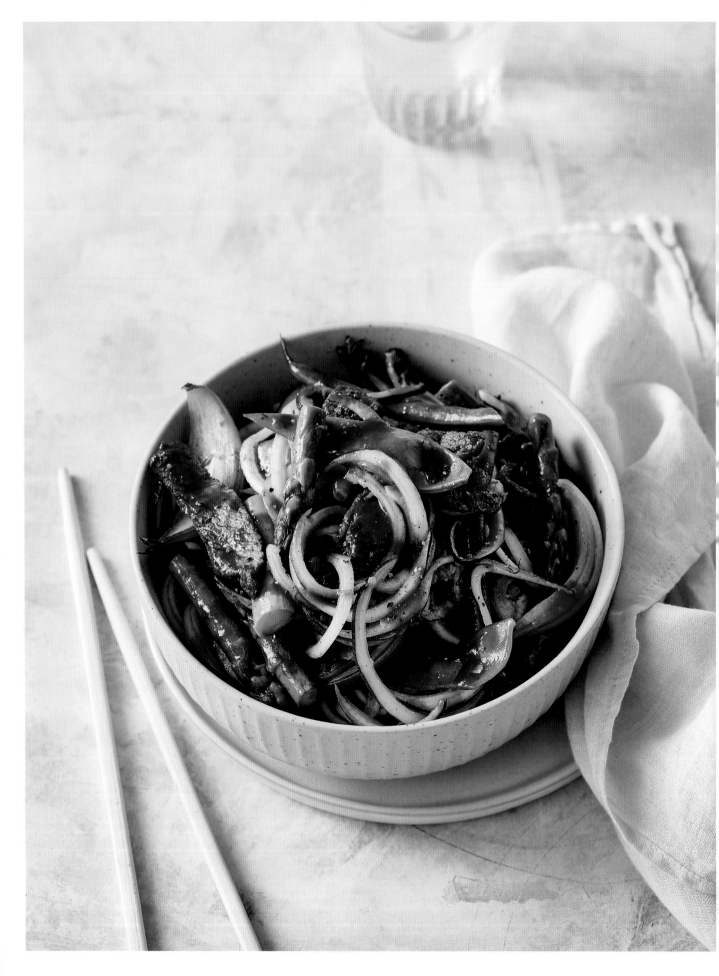

Five-spice beef stir-fry *and* hoisin greens

GRAMS CARB
14
PER SERVE

🍴 Serves 4 🕐 Preparation: 25 minutes
🌀 Cooking: 15 minutes ⏱ Difficulty: Low

1 red onion, cut into thin wedges
3 teaspoons Chinese five-spice powder
2 tablespoons sunflower oil
600 g lean rump steak, thinly sliced
3 bunches asparagus, trimmed and
   cut diagonally into 5 cm lengths
200 g baby green beans, trimmed
300 g snow peas, trimmed
2 x 250 g fresh zucchini noodles
   (see note)
2 tablespoons hoisin sauce

Combine the onion, five-spice powder and 1 tablespoon oil in a bowl. Add the steak and turn to combine and coat.

Heat a large non-stick wok over high heat. Add the beef in three batches and stir-fry for 2–3 minutes each or until just cooked and golden. Transfer to a bowl.

Heat the remaining oil in the wok. Add the asparagus, beans, snow peas, zucchini noodles, hoisin and 2 tablespoons water and stir-fry for 2–3 minutes or until just tender. Return all the beef and any resting juices to the wok and toss to combine.

Divide the stir-fry among bowls and serve immediately.

Note: You'll find fresh zucchini noodles in the fresh produce section at the supermarket. If unavailable, you can simply cut 4 zucchini into thin matchsticks and use as directed in the recipe.

UNITS PER SERVE

BREADS, CEREALS, LEGUMES, STARCHY VEGETABLES	DAIRY	LEAN MEAT, FISH, POULTRY, EGGS, TOFU	LOW-CARB VEGETABLES	MODERATE-CARB VEGETABLES	HEALTHY FATS
0	0	1.5	2	1	2

Roast beef *with* herb finishing sauce

🍽 Serves 4 🕐 Preparation: 30 minutes, plus 10 minutes resting time
🥘 Cooking: 35 minutes 🎩 Difficulty: Low

600 g lean beef topside roast
¼ cup (60 ml) olive oil
8 small zucchini, cut into thick chips
600 g parsnips, peeled and cut
   into thin chips
2 tablespoons rosemary leaves
100 g baby spinach leaves
100 g baby rocket leaves

HERB FINISHING SAUCE
1 teaspoon sweet paprika
½ cup (125 ml) red wine vinegar
¼ cup flat-leaf parsley leaves
2 tablespoons oregano leaves
100 g Greek-style yoghurt

Preheat the oven to 200°C (180°C fan-forced).

Place the beef in a large flameproof roasting tin and rub all over with 1 tablespoon oil. Add the zucchini, parsnip, rosemary leaves and remaining oil and toss to combine and coat. Season everything with freshly ground black pepper and roast for 25–30 minutes for medium or until the beef is cooked to your liking. Transfer the beef, zucchini and parsnip to a platter, cover loosely with foil and rest for 10 minutes.

To make the herb finishing sauce, add the paprika and vinegar to the roasting tin. Place the tin over medium heat and simmer, scraping off any bits caught on the base, for 3 minutes or until the vinegar has reduced by one-quarter. Pour the mixture into an upright blender, add the remaining ingredients and blend until smooth.

Carve the rested beef, then divide among serving plates, along with the vegetables. Drizzle over the herb finishing sauce and serve with the spinach and rocket leaves.

UNITS PER SERVE

BREADS, CEREALS, LEGUMES, STARCHY VEGETABLES	DAIRY	LEAN MEAT, FISH, POULTRY, EGGS, TOFU	LOW-CARB VEGETABLES	MODERATE-CARB VEGETABLES	HEALTHY FATS
0	>0.5	1.5	2	1	3

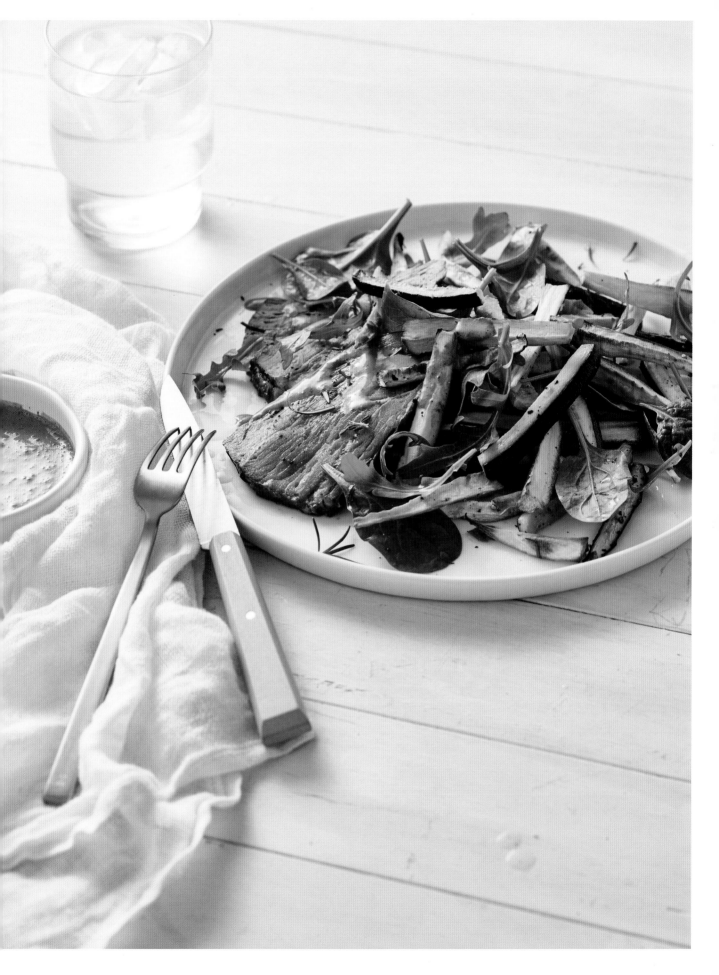

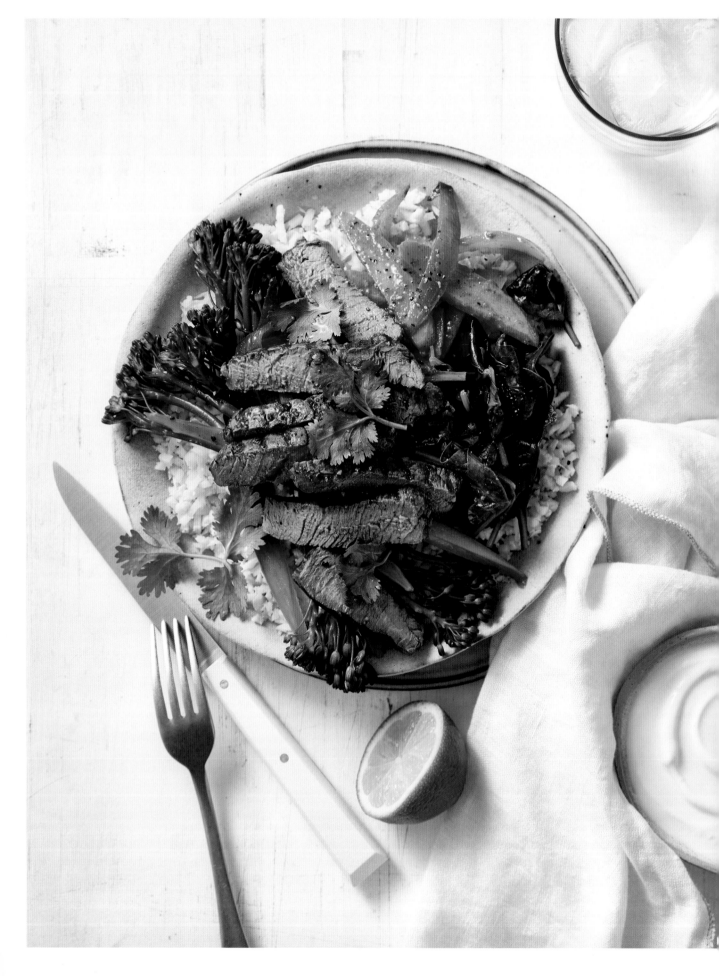

Beef fillet steaks
with korma vegetables

GRAMS CARB
13
PER SERVE

🍴 Serves 4 🕐 Preparation: 25 minutes, plus 3 minutes resting time
♨ Cooking: 10 minutes 🎓 Difficulty: Low

2 tablespoons korma curry paste
1 red onion, cut into thin wedges
1 carrot, halved lengthways,
   thinly sliced diagonally
3 bunches broccolini, trimmed
½ cup (125 ml) salt-reduced beef stock
150 g baby spinach leaves
100 g Greek-style yoghurt
4 x 150 g lean beef fillet steaks
500 g fresh cauliflower rice (see note)
½ cup coriander leaves

Heat the korma paste in a large deep non-stick frying pan over high heat. Add the onion and carrot and cook, stirring occasionally, for 3 minutes or until starting to soften. Reduce the heat to medium. Add the broccolini and stock and simmer, stirring occasionally, for 5 minutes or until almost tender. Add the spinach and stir until just wilted. Remove the pan from the heat, stir through the yoghurt and season with freshly ground black pepper.

Meanwhile, heat a chargrill pan over high heat. Season the steaks with freshly ground black pepper, then add to the pan and cook for 3–4 minutes each side for medium or until cooked to your liking. Transfer to serving plates, cover loosely with foil and leave to rest for 3 minutes before slicing.

Heat the cauliflower rice according to the packet instructions.

Divide the cauliflower rice among serving plates and top with the korma vegetables and steak. Sprinkle with the coriander and serve.

Note: You can find fresh cauliflower rice in the fresh produce section at your local supermarket. If unavailable, use the frozen variety instead.

UNITS PER SERVE

BREADS, CEREALS, LEGUMES, STARCHY VEGETABLES	DAIRY	LEAN MEAT, FISH, POULTRY, EGGS, TOFU	LOW-CARB VEGETABLES	MODERATE-CARB VEGETABLES	HEALTHY FATS
0	>0.5	1.5	2	1	2

Greek roasted lamb cutlets *and* veggies

GRAMS CARB 8 PER SERVE

🍴 Serves 4   🕐 Preparation: 25 minutes, plus 5 minutes resting time
🍲 Cooking: 25 minutes   ⏲ Difficulty: Low

150 g peeled, seeded pumpkin, thinly sliced

4 zucchini, thickly sliced into rounds

500 g cherry tomatoes

600 g lean French-trimmed lamb cutlets

2 tablespoons lamb dried herbs (see note)

2 tablespoons extra virgin olive oil

Finely grated zest and juice of 1 large lemon, plus extra lemon wedges to serve

1 cos lettuce, roughly chopped

80 g Greek feta, crumbled

80 g toasted slivered almonds

Preheat the oven to 200°C (180°C fan-forced) and line a large baking tray with baking paper.

Place the pumpkin, zucchini, tomatoes, lamb cutlets, dried herbs and 1 tablespoon oil on the prepared tray, tossing to combine and coat. Spread out in a single layer and roast for 20–25 minutes or until cooked and golden. Remove from the oven and rest for 5 minutes.

Meanwhile, whisk the lemon zest and juice with the remaining oil in a large bowl. Add the lettuce, feta and almonds and toss to combine.

Divide the lamb cutlets and vegetable mixture among plates and serve with the salad and lemon wedges.

Note: The lamb dried herbs seasoning mix is a combination of dried rosemary, garlic, thyme, oregano, mint, marjoram and basil and is readily available in the spice aisle at the supermarket. If unavailable, you can either make your own blend of all the herbs listed above or simply use 2 teaspoons each of dried rosemary, dried thyme, dried oregano and dried mint.

UNITS PER SERVE

BREADS, CEREALS, LEGUMES, STARCHY VEGETABLES	DAIRY	LEAN MEAT, FISH, POULTRY, EGGS, TOFU	LOW-CARB VEGETABLES	MODERATE-CARB VEGETABLES	HEALTHY FATS
0	1	1.5	2	0.5	4

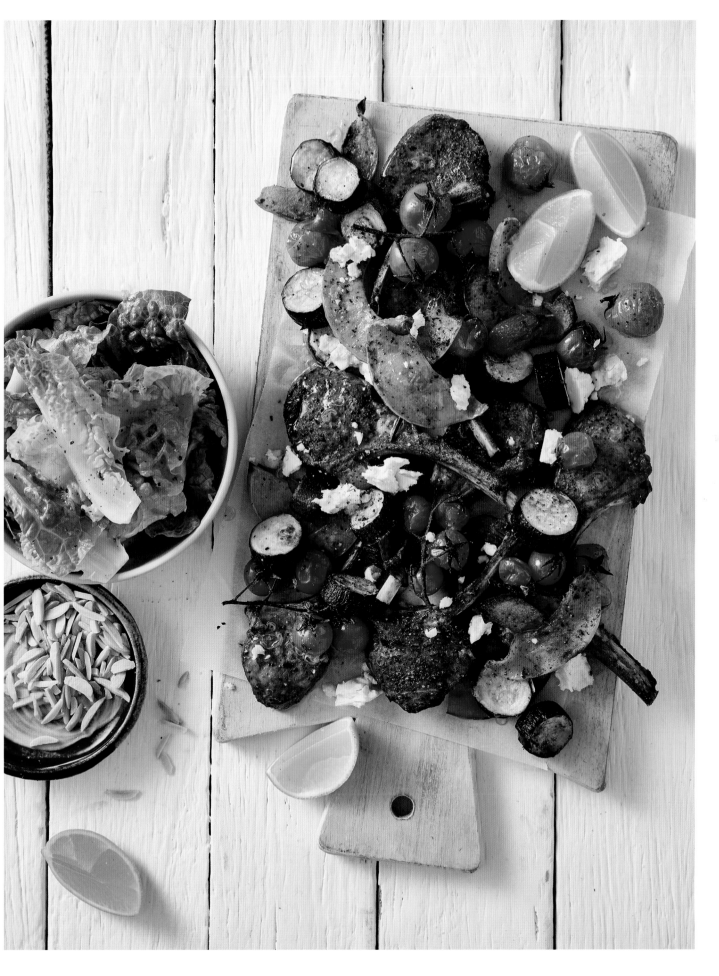

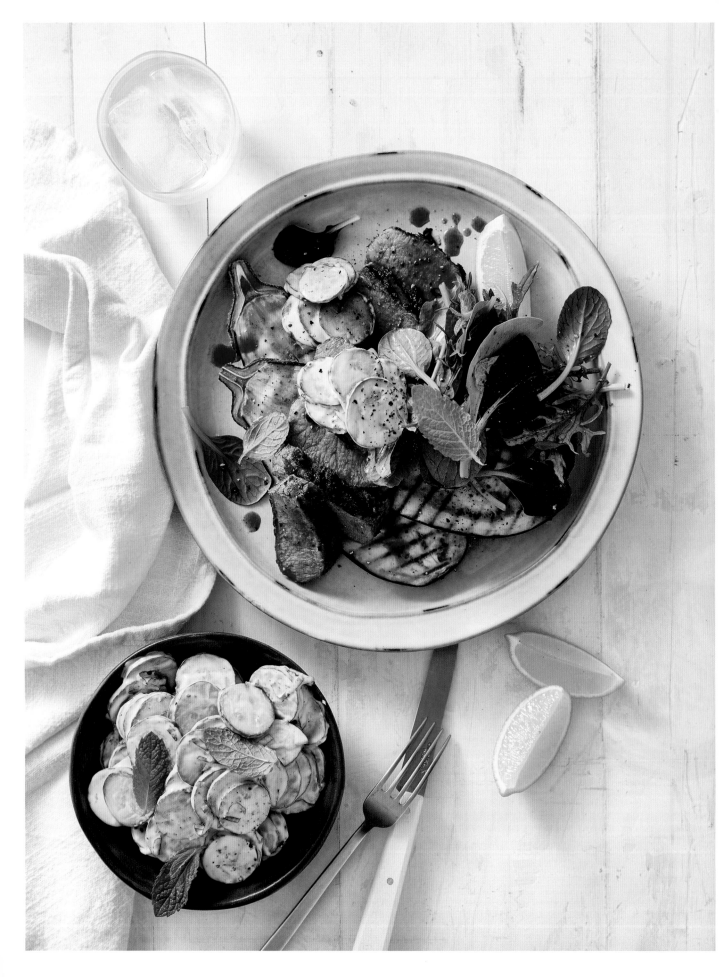

Vindaloo lamb *and* eggplant *with* raita

🍴 Serves 4   🕐 Preparation: 25 minutes, plus 5 minutes resting time
🍲 Cooking: 15 minutes   ⓢ Difficulty: Medium

2 tablespoons vindaloo curry paste
600 g lean lamb backstraps
2 eggplants, each cut lengthways
  into 4 thick slices
Olive oil spray, for cooking
200 g superleaf salad mix

RAITA
400 g Greek-style yoghurt
Finely grated zest and juice of 1 large
  lemon, plus extra lemon wedges
  to serve
8 Lebanese cucumbers, very thinly
  sliced into rounds
1 cup small mint leaves

To make the raita, combine all the ingredients in a large bowl. Season with freshly ground black pepper. Chill until required.

Preheat a barbecue chargrill plate to medium–high. Rub the curry paste all over the lamb. Lightly spray both sides of the eggplant slices with the olive oil, then season with freshly ground black pepper.

Chargrill the lamb and eggplant, turning once, for 10–12 minutes or until cooked and golden. Transfer the lamb to a board, cover loosely with foil and rest for 5 minutes before slicing thickly.

Divide the lamb, eggplant and salad mix among plates and serve with the raita and lemon wedges.

Note: The superleaf salad mix is a combination of spinach, chard, kale, red cabbage, beetroot and carrot and is readily available in the produce aisle at the supermarket. If unavailable, you can either make your own mix of the leaves listed above or simply use 100 g kale and 100 g baby spinach leaves.

UNITS PER SERVE

BREADS, CEREALS, LEGUMES, STARCHY VEGETABLES	DAIRY	LEAN MEAT, FISH, POULTRY, EGGS, TOFU	LOW-CARB VEGETABLES	MODERATE-CARB VEGETABLES	HEALTHY FATS
0	1	1.5	2	1	2

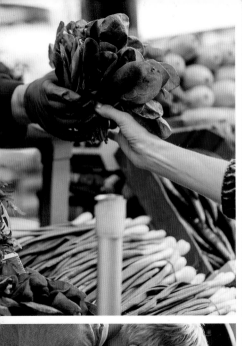
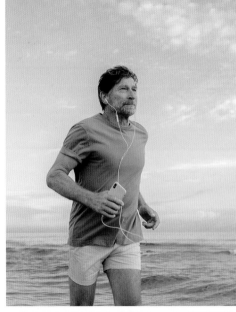
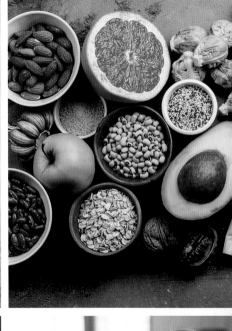
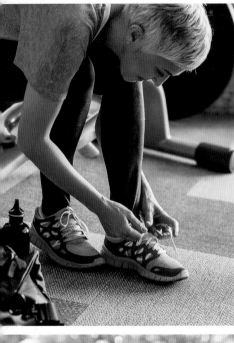

PART

5

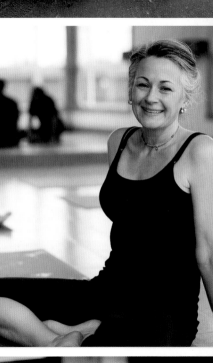
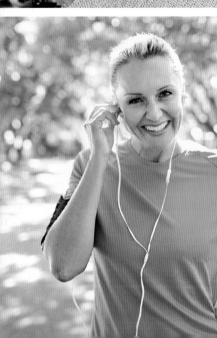
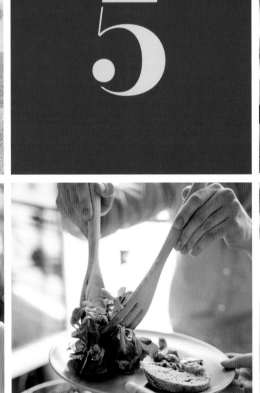
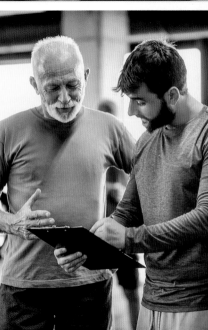

Using the

EXERCISE

PLAN

The CSIRO Low-carb Exercise Plan for Type 2 Diabetes

MODIFYING YOUR DIET IS INTEGRAL TO MANAGING YOUR WEIGHT, BLOOD GLUCOSE CONTROL AND METABOLIC RISK FACTORS; HOWEVER, BEING PHYSICALLY ACTIVE CAN PLAY AN EQUALLY IMPORTANT AND COMPLEMENTARY ROLE.

To achieve the most benefit from *The CSIRO Low-Carb Diabetes Diet & Lifestyle Solution*, you should also enjoy a physically active lifestyle.

Research clearly shows that having a high level of physical activity is one of the best predictors for sustaining a lower body weight over the long term. Evidence consistently shows that higher levels of physical activity are also associated with numerous health benefits that are achieved regardless of whether you lose weight – these include better blood glucose control; reduced risk of heart disease and premature death; lower blood pressure and blood cholesterol levels; improved mental health and performance; and reduced rates of some forms of cancer, depression and osteoporosis.

The two main ways to increase your physical activity are to participate in planned exercise, and to increase the amount of incidental physical activity that you do throughout the day.

▶ **Exercise** is a structured form of physical activity that is undertaken with a specific goal of sustaining or improving your health, fitness or wellbeing. An example of this is jogging or doing a gym workout.

▶ **Incidental physical activity** is activity that is done as part of general daily living, without a specific recreation, health or fitness goal. An example of this would be carrying heavy groceries, or walking up a flight of stairs rather than using an escalator or lift.

A comprehensive exercise program that provides the best overall mix of health benefits will include three types of exercise:

Exercise safety considerations

Before starting a new exercise program, it is a good idea to consult your healthcare team to ensure it is safe for you to do so, particularly if you have a pre-existing condition like high blood pressure, neuropathy, or any physical limitations. An accredited exercise physiologist is trained to be able to tailor the general exercise program provided in this book to meet your individual needs and abilities.

1 **Aerobic exercise**, also known as endurance exercise or cardiorespiratory fitness training (cardio). It involves sustained activities that use large muscle groups in a rhythmic manner, such as walking, swimming and cycling. This type of exercise helps to stabilise blood glucose and improves aerobic fitness, which reduces the risk of heart disease and premature death.

2 **Resistance training**, which is also known as strength or weight training. It consists of shorter, more intense activities that promote increases in muscle mass, strength, speed and power. These activities typically involve overloading the muscles with some kind of weight, such as your body weight or a dumbbell. This type of exercise increases muscle mass (or slows age-related muscle-mass loss), which enhances strength and metabolism, helps to stabilise blood glucose and increases bone strength. A higher muscle mass will also assist in maintaining a higher metabolism that helps you to burn more energy at rest, making it easier for you to maintain a healthier body weight.

3 **Flexibility and balance training.** Flexibility training is also commonly referred to as stretching. It involves stretching or repeatedly moving a joint through its complete range of motion. This type of exercise can increase (or prevent the loss of) joint range of motion, which makes the other types of exercise easier to perform, and improves general quality of life. Activities that maintain or improve balance (e.g. single leg stands) are important for older adults, particularly those with neuropathy, to help reduce the risk of falls. Most lower body and core resistance training exercises also improve balance. Yoga is also a great option for flexibility and balance training.

Your exercise plan that accompanies *The CSIRO Low-Carb Diabetes Diet & Lifestyle Solution* is based on these three components.

Aerobic EXERCISE PROGRAM

Your goal should be to achieve at least 150 minutes of moderate-intensity – or 75 minutes of vigorous-intensity – aerobic exercise per week (or an equivalent combination). Activities can range from brisk walking to jogging, cycling, rowing, aerobics, swimming and so on. Exercise should be performed in bouts of at least 10 minutes, with the aim of achieving about 30 minutes or more in total each day for most days of the week, and having no more than two consecutive days between bouts.

Rating of perceived exertion of exercise session	
0	Rest
1	Very, very easy
2	Easy
3	Moderate
4	Somewhat hard
5	Hard
6	–
7	Very hard
8	–
9	–
10	Maximum

Source: C Foster et al., 'A new approach to monitoring exercise training', *Journal of Strength and Conditioning Research*, 2001, vol. 15, no. 1, pp. 109–15.

Check your exercise intensity

For both the aerobic exercise and resistance training sessions, you can keep track of the relative intensity of your workout (i.e. the overall difficulty of the entire exercise session and how hard you worked) using a number from the adjacent table. A moderate-intensity workout, which you should be aiming for as a minimum, corresponds to a rating of 3.

Resistance TRAINING PROGRAM

Aim for at least two – more ideally, three – resistance training sessions each week, on non-consecutive days, with each session including 5–10 exercises involving major muscle groups (i.e. 2–4 upper-body exercises, 2–4 lower-body exercises, and 1–2 core exercises).

Try to perform 2–4 sets (batches of repetitions) of each exercise in your workout, allowing yourself 1–2 minutes rest between sets. Each set should consist of a sufficient number of repetitions of each exercise to induce muscle fatigue (i.e. the point at which you can no longer repeat the exercise without requiring a rest). Initially, you should aim to select a difficulty level (i.e. resistance or weight) that will allow you to perform 10–15 repetitions before you fatigue; once you become more established with the exercise program you can progress to a difficulty level that will cause fatigue within 8–10 repetitions.

As you become stronger, you will need to increase the difficulty (i.e. the resistance) of the exercise to continue to achieve the full benefits of the program. This is referred to as progressive overload. To minimise injury risk, take care to ensure that the technique of the exercise is not compromised as you increase the difficulty.

When performing these exercises, conduct each repetition at tempo 2–1–2 seconds (effort–hold–release phases). As an example, for the triceps kickback exercise on page 270, this would mean taking 2 seconds to lift the dumbbell, holding the dumbbell at the top for 1 second, then taking 2 seconds to return the dumbbell to the start position.

On the following pages you will find some exercise options that can be used to build a resistance training routine.

Remember your breathing!

While doing your resistance exercises, do not hold your breath. Breathe out during the effort phase, when the muscle is shortening under tension (e.g. when lifting a dumbbell), and breathe in during the release phase, when the muscle is lengthened under tension (e.g. when lowering the dumbbell).

Warm up AND cool down

Start each exercise session with a 5–10 minute warm-up that consists of gentle aerobic activities to prepare your body for exercise. For older adults, balance exercises such as single leg stands should also be incorporated into warm-ups on 2–3 days per week. Conclude each exercise session with a 5–10 minute cool-down, consisting of a range of flexibility exercises that stretch the major muscle groups, to bring your body back to a resting state.

Stay active: REDUCE SEDENTARY TIME

Remember to take every opportunity to be active. In addition to participating in a structured exercise program, try to take every opportunity to increase the amount of incidental physical activity you undertake, and to reduce the time spent sitting or lying down throughout the day. Some easy ways to do this are to walk up stairs instead of taking the lift, stand rather than sit when talking on the phone, take a short walk during your coffee break, or stand up during television advertisement breaks.

Research shows that independent of the amount of formal planned exercise you do, a high amount of sedentary time can present a separate risk factor for heart disease and type 2 diabetes.

UPPER BODY

Push-ups

FOR: Triceps (back upper arm), pectoral (chest)
WEIGHT: Bodyweight

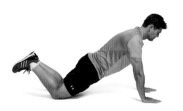
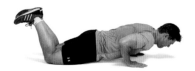

▶ **START POSITION:** Position your body facing the floor with your knees bent, back straight and your arms straight out in front of you. Your hands should be positioned slightly below shoulder level with your fingers pointed forwards, and spaced a little further than shoulder width apart.
▶ **ACTION 1:** Lower your body, pivoting from your knees, with your elbows slightly out, until your chest is an inch or two above the floor.
▶ **ACTION 2:** Push your torso away from the ground until your arms are straight.

EASIER VARIATION: Perform the exercise with your hands against the wall while standing, instead of laying on the floor, using your feet as a pivot point.
ADVANCED VARIATION: Straighten your legs, and use your toes as a pivot point.

Triceps kickback

FOR: Triceps (back upper arm)
WEIGHT: Dumbbell

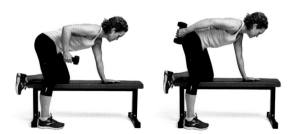

▶ **START POSITION:** Stand side-on to the right-hand side of a bench, holding a dumbbell in your right hand with your palm facing in. Lean forward at the waist and position your left knee and left hand on the bench. Bend your right elbow and raise your upper arm so it is parallel to the floor. Your forearm should remain pointing down.
▶ **ACTION 1:** Keeping your upper arm still and your elbow close to your torso, straighten your arm behind you until your entire arm is parallel to the floor, and the front end of the dumbbell points towards the floor.
▶ **ACTION 2:** Slowly bring the dumbbell back to the start position.
▶ **ACTION 3:** Perform all right side repetitions within a set first before switching to the left side. A complete left and right side sequence of repetitions equals one set.

Bench dips

FOR: Triceps (back upper arm), deltoid (shoulders)
WEIGHT: Bodyweight

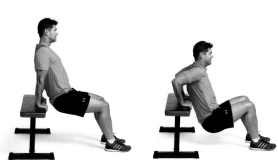
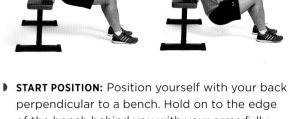

▶ **START POSITION:** Position yourself with your back perpendicular to a bench. Hold on to the edge of the bench behind you with your arms fully extended, hands spaced a little further than shoulder width apart. Your legs should be extended forward with a slight bend in the knee.

▶ **ACTION 1:** Slowly lower your body by bending at the elbows, until you lower yourself far enough to where there is an angle slightly smaller than 90 degrees between your upper arm and forearm. Try to keep your elbows over your hands.

▶ **ACTION 2:** Lift yourself back to the start position.

EASIER VARIATION: Perform the exercise on the floor without a bench. Sitting on the floor with your hands flat behind you (fingers pointing forward), slowly lower your body weight backward and over your hands by bending at the elbows, then push yourself up to the start position.

ADVANCED VARIATION 1: Place your legs on top of another flat bench in front of you to make the exercise more challenging.

ADVANCED VARIATION 2: Have a partner place a weight plate on top of your lap, asking your partner to ensure that the weight stays there throughout the movement.

Bicep curl

FOR: Biceps (front upper arm)
WEIGHT: Dumbbells

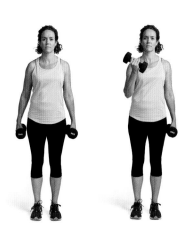

▶ **START POSITION:** Stand upright with your arms by your side and a dumbbell in each hand. Your elbows should be close to your torso and your palms should be facing the side of your thighs.

▶ **ACTION 1:** While maintaining a stationary upper arm, lift the dumbbell in your right hand as you rotate the palm of the hand upwards. Continue to lift the dumbbell until it is at shoulder level.

▶ **ACTION 2:** Slowly bring the dumbbell back to the start position.

▶ **ACTION 3:** Repeat the movement on the left side. A complete left and right side sequence equals one repetition.

UPPER BODY

Shoulder lateral raises

FOR: Deltoid (shoulder)
WEIGHT: Dumbbells

Dumbbell upright row

FOR: Trapezius (back)
WEIGHT: Dumbbells

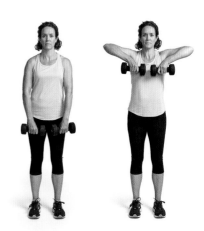

▶ **START POSITION:** Stand upright with your arms by your side and a dumbbell in each hand. Your elbows should be close to your torso, and your palms should be facing the sides of your thighs. Perform half a bicep curl (see page 271), bending your elbows so they are flexed at a 90-degree angle.
▶ **ACTION 1:** Keep your torso still and bring your upper arms outwards and upwards while maintaining the 90-degree elbow bend. Do not allow your shoulders to rotate. Continue to lift up until your arms are parallel to the floor.
▶ **ACTION 2:** Slowly lower the dumbbells back down to the starting position.

EASIER VARIATION: This exercise can also be performed sitting down.
ADVANCED VARIATION: Conduct the exercise with straight arms, taking the dumbbells from your sides straight out to shoulder-height.

▶ **START POSITION:** Stand upright with your arms pointing down in front of you and a dumbbell in each hand. Your palms should be facing the front of your thighs.
▶ **ACTION 1:** Keep your torso still and use your shoulders to lift both dumbbells up simultaneously until they nearly touch your chin, keeping them close to your body the entire time. As you lift up, your elbows should remain higher than your hands.
▶ **ACTION 2:** Slowly lower the dumbbells back down to the starting position.

Front dumbbell raise

FOR: Deltoid (shoulder), trapezius (back)
WEIGHT: Dumbbells

Bent-over two-dumbbell row

FOR: Trapezius and rhomboids (back)
WEIGHT: Dumbbells

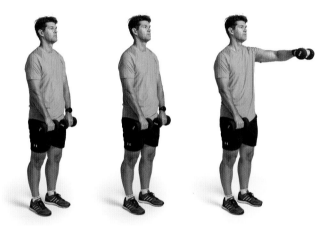

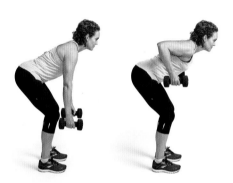

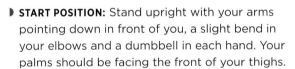

▶ **START POSITION:** Stand upright with your arms pointing down in front of you, a slight bend in your elbows and a dumbbell in each hand. Your palms should be facing the front of your thighs.

▶ **ACTION 1:** Keep your torso still and bring your right arm upwards in front of you while maintaining a slight bend in your elbow. Do not rotate your shoulder during the lift. Continue to lift up until your arm is parallel to the floor and the dumbbell is at shoulder height.

▶ **ACTION 2:** Lower the dumbbell back down slowly to the starting position as you simultaneously lift the left dumbbell up. A complete left and right side sequence equals one repetition.

▶ **START POSITION:** Stand upright with your knees bent slightly. Bend forward at the waist so you are leaning over your feet, keeping your spine in its natural (neutral) curvature. Hold a dumbbell in each hand (palms facing each other), with your arms hanging straight down in front of you. Keep your head up, facing forward.

▶ **ACTION 1:** Keep your torso stationary and lift both dumbbells simultaneously up to your side, squeezing your shoulder blades together.

▶ **ACTION 2:** Slowly lower the dumbbells back to the start position.

CAUTION! This exercise is not recommended for people with back problems.

LOWER BODY

Deadlift

FOR: Hamstrings (back upper leg)
WEIGHT: Dumbbells

Squats

FOR: Quads (front upper leg), glutes (buttocks)
WEIGHT: Bodyweight

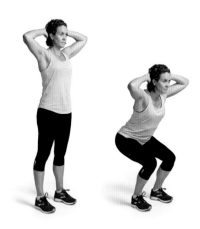

▶ **START POSITION:** Stand upright with your arms pointing down in front of you and a dumbbell in each hand. Your palms should be facing the front of your thighs, and your weight should be on your heels.

▶ **ACTION 1:** Keeping your back straight, your bodyweight on your heels, and your arms down, bend at the hips to push your butt backwards as far as possible, keeping your torso and stomach tight. Your knees should bend just a small amount, and you should keep your chest up and your spine in its natural (neutral) curvature.

▶ **ACTION 2:** Slowly bring the hips forward to return to the start position.

▶ **START POSITION:** Stand upright with your feet shoulder width apart. Place your hands behind your head.

▶ **ACTION 1:** Flex your knees and hips so you are sitting back, keeping your weight on your heels. Keep your head and chest up high, and your butt out during the movement. Squat down to as low as you are able to — like you are going to sit on a chair.

▶ **ACTION 2:** Reverse the motion, coming back up to standing position.

ADVANCED VARIATION: Hold a dumbbell in each hand by your side, with your palms facing the side of your thighs.

Forward lunge

FOR: Quads (front upper leg), glutes (buttocks)
WEIGHT: Bodyweight

Glute kickbacks

FOR: Glutes (buttocks)
WEIGHT: Bodyweight

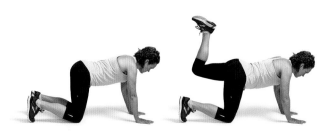

▶ **START POSITION:** Stand upright with your feet shoulder width apart. Place your hands on your hips.

▶ **ACTION 1:** While maintaining an upright posture, take a moderate step forward with your right foot. Descend your hips until your left knee approaches the floor without touching it. Your right knee should bend to approximately 90 degrees and should not go past your toes (take a slightly larger step to avoid this if required).

▶ **ACTION 2:** Push back up from your right foot, bringing it back to the start position.

▶ **ACTION 3:** Repeat the movement with the left foot stepping forward. A complete left and right side sequence equals one repetition.

ADVANCED VARIATION: Hold a dumbbell in each hand by your side, with your palms facing the side of your thighs.

▶ **START POSITION:** Kneel on the floor with your knees bent at 90 degrees, your waist bent slightly forward, your spine in its natural (neutral) curvature and your arms out in front of you. Your hands should be positioned on the floor shoulder width apart, and your head facing down at the ground.

▶ **ACTION 1:** Lift your left leg, while maintaining the 90-degree knee bend, until your upper leg is parallel with the ground.

▶ **ACTION 2:** Lower your leg back to the start position.

▶ **ACTION 3:** Repeat the movement with the right leg. A complete left and right side sequence equals one repetition.

LOWER BODY

Calf raises

FOR: Calves (lower leg)
WEIGHT: Bodyweight

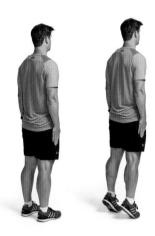

▶ **START POSITION:** Stand upright with your feet shoulder width apart, supporting your weight on the balls of your feet. Your feet should be pointing straight forwards. Have your arms by your side, with your palms facing the side of your thighs. If you are having trouble balancing, support yourself by holding onto a doorframe with one hand.
▶ **ACTION 1:** Raise your heels off the floor by contracting your calf muscles (pointing your feet down).
▶ **ACTION 2:** Lower yourself slowly back down until your heels contact the ground.

ADVANCED VARIATION 1: Have your arms by your side and a dumbbell in each hand (palms facing the side of your thighs). If you are having trouble balancing, use one dumbbell only, and support yourself by holding onto a doorframe with your free hand.
ADVANCED VARIATION 2: To increase the range of motion, stand with your toes and the balls of your feet on a sturdy wooden board or step about 5–10 cm thick, and your heels extending off and touching the ground.

Bridge

FOR: Glutes (buttocks), hamstrings (back upper leg)
WEIGHT: Bodyweight

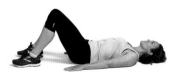

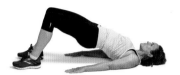

▶ **START POSITION:** Lie down on the floor, on your back, with your knees bent at approximately 90 degrees, and your feet flat on the floor and shoulder width apart. Your arms should be loosely by your side, with palms facing the floor for stability.
▶ **ACTION 1:** While keeping your back straight, lift your hips upwards off the floor by pushing through your heels until your knees, hips and shoulders are in a straight line.
▶ **ACTION 2:** Slowly return to the start position.

ADVANCED VARIATION: Perform this exercise with a single leg at a time (i.e. lift one foot off the ground). If that variation also becomes easy, hold a weight plate on top of your lap while you perform the exercise.

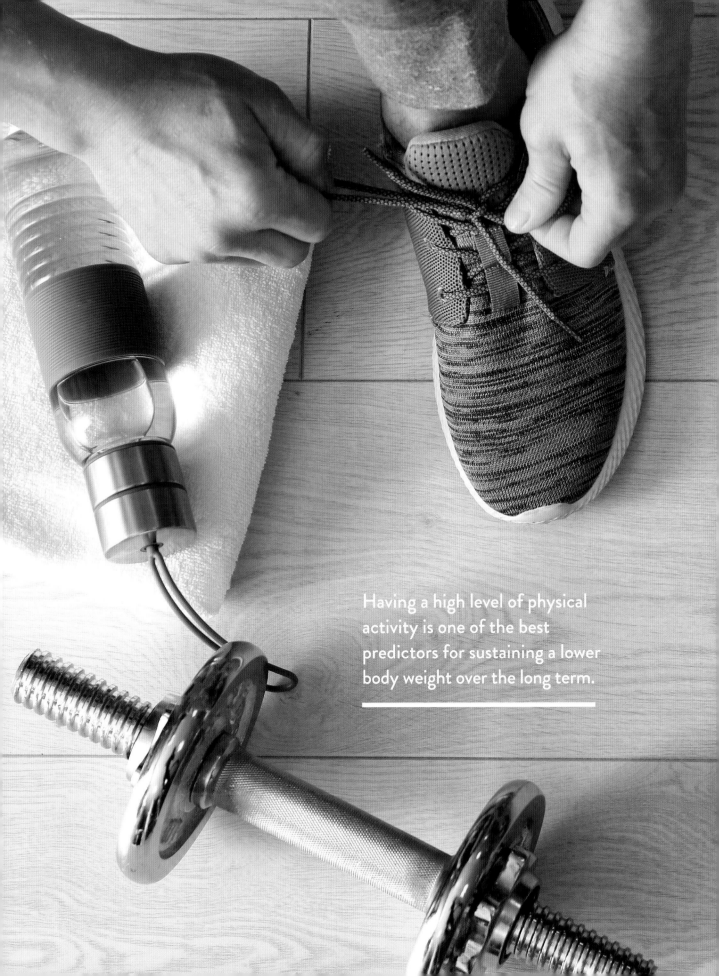

Having a high level of physical activity is one of the best predictors for sustaining a lower body weight over the long term.

CORE

Sit-ups

FOR: Abdominals (stomach)
WEIGHT: Bodyweight

Bicycle crunches

FOR: Abdominal obliques (stomach)
WEIGHT: Bodyweight

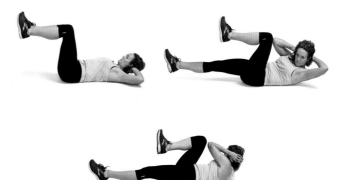

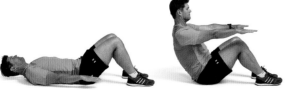

▶ **START POSITION:** Lie down on the floor, on your back, with your knees bent 90 degrees, and your feet flat on the floor, with your toes held under something that will not move (or a partner holding your feet to the floor). Your arms should be by your side, raised slightly off the floor and pointing towards your feet.

▶ **ACTION 1:** Keeping your feet and butt on the floor, and arms parallel to the floor, raise your shoulder blades and torso up off the floor, coming up to your knees as far as you can. Take care not to strain your neck forward as you raise.

▶ **ACTION 2:** Slowly lower your torso and shoulder blades back to the floor.

ADVANCED VARIATION: Keep your feet flat on the floor without having them held. Crossing your arms in front of your chest or placing your hands behind your head will progressively increase the difficulty.

▶ **START POSITION:** Lie on your back, on the floor. Place your hands behind your head, with your elbows out to the side. Bend your knees and waist to 90 degrees, so that your lower legs are raised and parallel to the floor. Lift your shoulder blades into the 'crunch' position.

▶ **ACTION 1:** Perform a cycle pedal motion, kicking forward with the right leg and bringing in the knee of the left leg. As your left knee comes up, bring your right elbow across to it, by crunching to the left.

▶ **ACTION 2:** Continue the cycle motion with your legs, kicking forward with the left leg and bringing in the knee of the right leg. As your right knee comes up, bring your left elbow across to it by crunching to the right.

▶ **ACTION 3:** A complete left and right side sequence equals one repetition.

Plank

Opposite arm/leg raise

FOR: Abdominals (stomach)
WEIGHT: Bodyweight

FOR: Deltoids (shoulder), abdominals (stomach), glutes (butt)
WEIGHT: Bodyweight

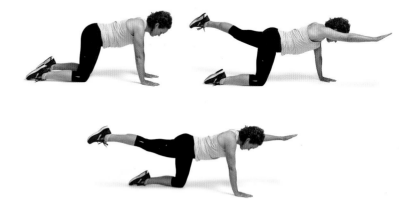

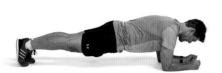

▶ **START POSITION:** Position your body face down to the floor. Your upper arms should be pointing straight down to the floor, with your elbows shoulder width apart and bent at 90 degrees, so your forearms are flat on the floor, facing forward in an inverted 'V', with your hands in front of your face. You should be looking at the floor, and your weight should be supported entirely on your toes and your forearms. Your body should be in a straight line, without your butt sticking up.

▶ **ACTION:** Keep your body straight and hold this position for at least 30 seconds.

EASY VARIATION: Drop your knees to the ground and perform the exercise in this position.
ADVANCED VARIATION: Increase the length of time you hold the plank position and push forward further from your toes.

▶ **START POSITION:** Position yourself on all fours with your back straight, knees below your hips, hands below your shoulders, and arms straight.

▶ **ACTION 1:** Reach your right arm out in front of you, while simultaneously extending your left leg out behind you. Your right arm, back and left leg should form a straight line.

▶ **ACTION 2:** Slowly return to the start position.

▶ **ACTION 3:** Repeat on the opposite side, raising your left arm and right leg. A complete left and right side sequence equals one repetition.

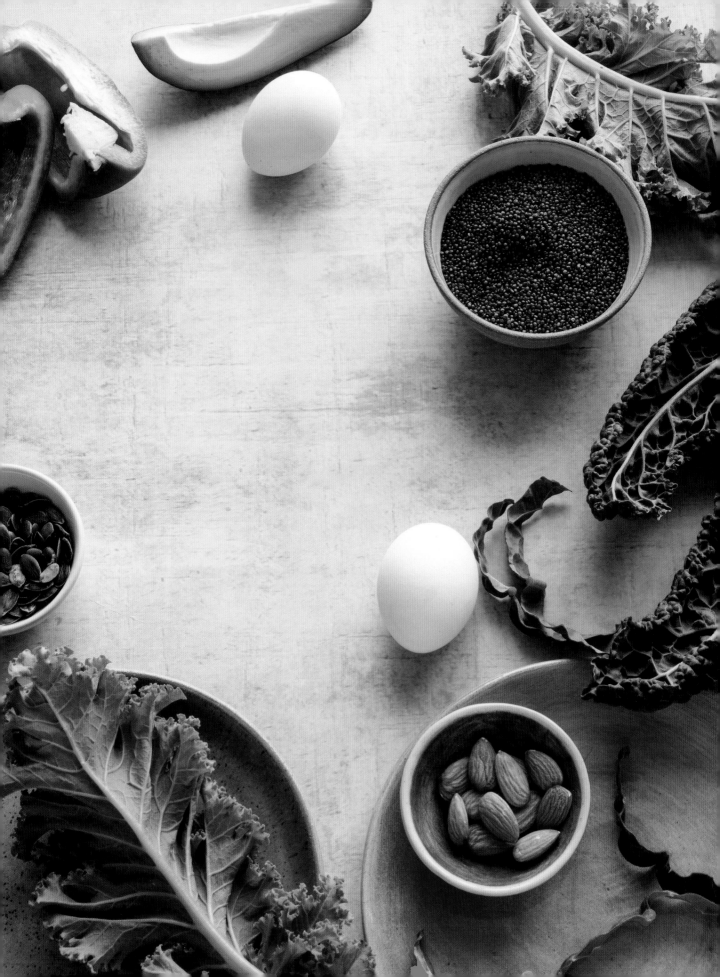

References

American Diabetes Association. 'Facilitating behavior change and well-being to improve health outcomes: standards of medical care in diabetes – 2020.' *Diabetes Care.* 2020 Jan; 43(Supplement 1): S48-S65.

Aucott L, Poobalan A, Smith WC, Avenell A, Jung R, Broom J, Grant AM. 'Weight loss in obese diabetic and non-diabetic individuals and long-term diabetes outcomes – a systematic review.' *Diabetes Obes Metab.* 2004;6(2):85-94.

Barnosky AR, Hoddy KK, Unterman TG, Varady KA. 'Intermittent fasting vs daily calorie restriction for type 2 diabetes prevention: a review of human findings.' *Transl Res.* Oct 2014;164(4):302-311.

Bommer C, Sagalova V, Heesemann E, Manne-Goehler J, Atun R, Barnighausen T, Davies J, Vollmer S. 'Global economic burden of diabetes in adults: projections from 2015 to 2030.' *Diabetes Care.* May 2018;41(5):963-970.

Brennan IM, Luscombe-Marsh ND, Seimon RV, Otto B, Horowitz M, Wishart JM, Feinle-Bisset C. 'Effects of fat, protein, and carbohydrate and protein load on appetite, plasma cholecystokinin, peptide YY, and ghrelin, and energy intake in lean and obese men.' *Am J Physiol Gastrointest Liver Physiol.* 2012;303(1):G129-40.

British Dietetic Association (2018). 'Low carbohydrate diets for the management of Type 2 Diabetes in adults.' https://www.bda.uk.com/improvinghealth/healthprofessionals/policy_statements/policy_statement_-_low_carbohydrate_diets_t2_diabetes

Brinkworth GD, Buckley JD, Noakes M, Clifton PM. 'Renal function following long-term weight loss in individuals with abdominal obesity on a very-low-carbohydrate diet vs high-carbohydrate diet.' *J Am Diet Assoc;*110(4):633-8.

Brinkworth GD, Luscombe-Marsh ND, Thompson CH, Noakes M, Buckley JD, Wittert G, Wilson CJ. 'Long-term effects of very low-carbohydrate and high-carbohydrate weight-loss diets on psychological health in obese adults with type 2 diabetes: randomized controlled trial.' *J Intern Med.* 2016;280(4):388-97.

Brinkworth GD, Noakes M, Buckley JD, Keogh JB, Clifton PM. 'Long-term effects of a very-low-carbohydrate weight loss diet compared with an isocaloric low-fat diet after 12 mo.' *Am J Clin Nutr.* 2009;90(1):23-32.

Brinkworth GD, Wycherley TP, Noakes M, Buckley JD, Clifton PM. 'Long-term effects of a very-low-carbohydrate weight-loss diet and an isocaloric low-fat diet on bone health in obese adults.' *Nutrition.* 2016;32(9):1033-6.

Carter S, Clifton PM, Keogh JB. 'Effect of intermittent compared with continuous energy restricted diet on glycemic control in patients with type 2 diabetes: a randomized noninferiority trial.' *JAMA Netw Open.* Jul 6 2018;1(3):e180756.

Cavalot F, Petrelli A, Traversa M, Bonomo K, Fiora E, Conti M, Anfossi G, Costa G, Trovati M. 'Postprandial blood glucose is a stronger predictor of cardiovascular events than fasting blood glucose in type 2 diabetes mellitus, particularly in women: lessons from the San Luigi Gonzaga Diabetes Study.' *J Clin Endocrinol Metab.* 2006;91(3):813-9.

Chang CR, BFrancois ME, Little JP. 'Restricting carbohydrates at breakfast is sufficient to reduce 24-hour exposure to postprandial hyperglycemia and improve glycemic variability.' *Am J Clin Nutr.* 2019;109:1302-1309.

Diabetes Australia (2018). 'Position Statement: Low carbohydrate eating for people with diabetes.' https://static.diabetesaustralia.com.au/s/fileassets/diabetes-australia/dbd70857-a834-45b0-b6f1-ea2582bbe5c7.pdf

Diabetes UK (2017). 'Position statement: Low-carb diets for people living with diabetes.' https://www.diabetes.org.uk/resources-s3/2017-09/low-carb-diets-position-statement-May-2017.pdf

Farnsworth E, Luscombe ND, Noakes M, Wittert G, Argyiou E, Clifton PM. 'Effect of a high-protein, energy-restricted diet on body composition, glycemic control, and lipid concentrations in overweight and obese hyperinsulinemic men and women.' *Am J Clin Nutr.* 2003;78(1):31-9.

Faulconbridge LF, Wadden TA, Rubin RR, Wing RR, Walkup MP, Fabricatore AN, Coday M, Van Dorsten B, Mount DL, Ewing LJ. 'One-year changes in symptoms of depression and weight in overweight/obese individuals with type 2 diabetes in the Look AHEAD study.' *Obesity (Silver Spring).* 2012;20(4):783-93.

Foster GD, Wyatt HR, Hill JO, McGuckin BG, Brill C, Mohammed BS, Szapary PO, Rader DJ, Edman JS, Klein S. 'A randomized trial of a low-carbohydrate diet for obesity.' *N Engl J Med.* 2003;348(21):2082-90.

Francois ME, Myette-Cote E, Bammert TD, Durrer C, Neudorf H, DeSouza CA, Little JP. 'Carbohydrate restriction with postmeal walking effectively mitigates postprandial hyperglycemia and improves endothelial function in type 2 diabetes.' *Am J Physiol Heart Circ Physiol.* Jan 1 2018;314(1):H105-H113.

Fuentes F, Lopez-Miranda J, Sanchez E, Sanchez F, Paez J, Paz-Rojas E, Marin C, Gomez P, Jimenez-Pereperez J, Ordovas JM, Perez-Jimenez F. 'Mediterranean and low-fat diets improve endothelial function in hypercholesterolemic men'. *Ann Intern Med.* 2001;134(12):1115-9.

Gannon MC, Nuttall FQ, Saeed A, Jordan K, Hoover H. 'An increase in dietary protein improves the blood glucose response in persons with type 2 diabetes.' *Am J Clin Nutr.* 2003;78(4):734-41.

Gardner CD, Kiazand A, Alhassan S, Kim S, Stafford RS, Balise RR, Kraemer HC, King AC. 'Comparison of the Atkins, Zone, Ornish, and LEARN diets for change in weight and related risk factors among overweight premenopausal women: the A TO Z Weight Loss Study: a randomized trial.' *JAMA.* 2007;297(9):969-77.

Gentilcore D, Chaikomin R, Jones KL, Russo A, Feinle-Bisset C, Wishart JM, Rayner CK, Horowitz M. 'Effects of fat on gastric emptying of and the glycemic, insulin, and incretin responses to a carbohydrate meal in type 2 diabetes.' *J Clin Endocrinol Metab.* 2006;91(6):2062-7.

Gibson AA, Seimon RV, Lee CM, Ayre J, Franklin J, Markovic TP, Caterson ID, Sainsbury A. 'Do ketogenic diets really suppress appetite? A systematic review and meta-analysis.' *Obes Rev.* 2015;16(1):64-76.

Gjuladin-Hellon T, Davies IG, Penson P, Amiri Baghbadorani R. 'Effects of carbohydrate-restricted diets on low-density lipoprotein cholesterol levels in overweight and obese adults: a systematic review and meta-analysis.' *Nutr Rev.* Mar 1 2019;77(3):161-180.

Harvey C, Schofield GM, Zinn C, Thornley SJ, Crofts C, Merien FLR. 'Low-carbohydrate diets differing in carbohydrate restriction improve cardiometabolic and anthropometric markers in healthy adults: A randomised clinical trial.' *PeerJ.* 2019;7:e6273.

Hession M, Rolland C, Kulkarni U, Wise A, Broom J. 'Systematic review of randomized controlled trials of low-carbohydrate vs. low-fat/low-calorie diets in the management of obesity and its comorbidities.' *Obes Rev.* Jan 2009;10(1):36-50.

Jesudason DR, Pedersen E, Clifton PM. 'Weight-loss diets in people with type 2 diabetes and renal disease: a randomized controlled trial of the effect of different dietary protein amounts.' *Am J Clin Nutr.* 2013;98(2):494-501.

Keogh JB, Grieger JA, Noakes M, Clifton PM. 'Flow-mediated dilatation is impaired by a high-saturated fat diet but not by a high-carbohydrate diet.' *Arterioscler Thromb Vasc Biol.* 2005;25(6):1274-9.

Klonoff DC, Ahn D, Drincic A. 'Continuous glucose monitoring: A review of the technology and clinical use.' *Diabetes Res Clin Pract.* Nov 2017;133:178-192.

Kodama S, Saito K, Tanaka S, Maki M, Yachi Y, Sato M, Sugawara A, Totsuka K, Shimano H, Ohashi Y, Yamada N, Sone H. 'Influence of fat and carbohydrate proportions on the metabolic profile in patients with type 2 diabetes: a meta-analysis.' *Diabetes Care.* May 2009;32(5):959-965.

Krauss RM, Blanche PJ, Rawlings RS, Fernstrom HS, Williams PT. 'Separate effects of reduced carbohydrate intake and weight loss on atherogenic dyslipidemia.' *Am J Clin Nutr.* 2006;83(5):1025-31.

Leidy HJ, Clifton PM, Astrup A, Wycherley TP, Westerterp-Plantenga MS, Luscombe-Marsh ND, Woods SC, Mattes RD. 'The role of protein in weight loss and maintenance.' *Am J Clin Nutr.* 2015.

Lean MEJ, Leslie WS, Barnes AC, Brosnahan N, Thom G, McCombie L, Peters C, Zhyzhneuskaya S, Al-Mrabeh A, Hollingsworth KG, Rodrigues AM, Rehackova L, Adamson AJ, Sniehotta FF, Mathers JC, Ross HM, McIlvenna Y, Welsh P, Kean S, Ford I, McConnachie A, Messow CM, Sattar N, Taylor R. 'Durability of a primary care-led weight-management intervention for remission of type 2 diabetes: 2-year results of the DiRECT open-label, cluster-randomised trial.' *Lancet Diabetes Endocrinol.* May 2019;7(5):344-355.

Look ARG, Pi-Sunyer X, Blackburn G, Brancati FL, Bray GA, Bright R, Clark JM, Curtis JM, Espeland MA, Foreyt JP, Graves K, et al. 'Reduction in weight and cardiovascular disease risk factors in individuals with type 2 diabetes: one-year results of the look AHEAD trial.' *Diabetes Care.* 2007;30(6):1374-83.

Ma J, Stevens JE, Cukier K, Maddox AF, Wishart JM, Jones KL, Clifton PM, Horowitz M, Rayner CK. 'Effects of a protein preload on gastric emptying, glycemia, and gut hormones after a carbohydrate meal in diet-controlled type 2 diabetes.' *Diabetes Care.* 2009;32(9):1600-2.

MacLeod J, Franz MJ, Handu D, Gradwell E, Brown C, Evert A, Reppert A, Robinson M. 'Academy of nutrition and dietetics nutrition practice guideline for type 1 and type 2 diabetes in adults: nutrition intervention evidence reviews and recommendations.' *J Acad Nutr Diet.* Oct 2017;117(10):1637-1658.

Mayer SB, Jeffreys AS, Olsen MK, McDuffie JR, Feinglos MN, Yancy WS, Jr. 'Two diets with different haemoglobin A1c and antiglycaemic medication effects despite similar weight loss in type 2 diabetes.' *Diabetes Obes Metab.* 2014;16(1):90-3.

Meng Y, Bai H, Wang S, Li Z, Wang Q, Chen L. 'Efficacy of low carbohydrate diet for type 2 diabetes mellitus management: A systematic review and meta-analysis of randomized controlled trials.' *Diabetes Res Clin Pract.* Sep 2017;131:124-131.

Mensink RP, Zock PL, Kester AD, Katan MB. 'Effects of dietary fatty acids and carbohydrates on the ratio of serum total to HDL cholesterol and on serum lipids and apolipoproteins: a meta-analysis of 60 controlled trials'. *Am J Clin Nutr.* 2003;77(5):1146-55.

Myette-Cote E, Durrer C, Neudorf H, Bammert TD, Botezelli JD, Johnson JD, DeSouza CA, Little JP. 'The effect of a short-term low-carbohydrate, high-fat diet with or without postmeal walks on glycemic control and inflammation in type 2 diabetes: a randomized trial.' *Am J Physiol Regul Integr Comp Physiol.* Dec 1 2018;315(6):R1210-R1219.

Nordmann AJ, Nordmann A, Briel M, Keller U, Yancy WS, Jr., Brehm BJ, Bucher HC. 'Effects of low-carbohydrate vs low-fat diets on weight loss and cardiovascular risk factors: a meta-analysis of randomized controlled trials.' *Arch Intern Med.* 2006;166(3):285-93.

Murdoch C, Unwin D, Cavan D, Cucuzzella M, Patel M. 'Adapting diabetes medication for low carbohydrate management of type 2 diabetes: a practical guide.' *Br J Gen Pract.* Jul 2019;69(684):360-361.

Olczuk D, Priefer R. 'A history of continuous glucose monitors (CGMs) in self-monitoring of diabetes mellitus.' *Diabetes Metab Syndr.* Apr–Jun 2018;12(2):181-187.

Pan B, Ge L, Xun YQ, Chen YJ, Gao CY, Han X, Zuo LQ, Shan HQ, Yang KH, Ding GW, Tian JH. 'Exercise training modalities in patients with type 2 diabetes mellitus: a systematic review and network meta-analysis.' *Int J Behav Nutr Phys Act.* Jul 25 2018;15(1):72.

Parker B, Noakes M, Luscombe N, Clifton P. 'Effect of a high-protein, high-monounsaturated fat weight loss diet on glycemic control and lipid levels in type 2 diabetes.' *Diabetes Care.* 2002;25(3):425-30.

Rallidis LS, Lekakis J, Kolomvotsou A, Zampelas A, Vamvakou G, Efstathiou S, Dimitriadis G, Raptis SA, Kremastinos DT. 'Close adherence to a Mediterranean diet improves endothelial function in subjects with abdominal obesity.' *Am J Clin Nutr.* 2009;90(2):263-8.

Riccardi G, Giacco R, Rivellese AA. 'Dietary fat, insulin sensitivity and the metabolic syndrome.' *Clin Nutr.* 2004;23(4):447-56.

Rock CL, Flatt SW, Pakiz B, Taylor KS, Leone AF, Brelje K, Heath DD, Quintana EL, Sherwood NE. 'Weight loss, glycemic control, and cardiovascular disease risk factors in response to differential diet composition in a weight loss program in type 2 diabetes: a randomized controlled trial.' *Diabetes Care.* 2014;37(6):1573-80.

Sainsbury E, Kizirian NV, Partridge SR, Gill T, Colagiuri S, Gibson AA. 'Effect of dietary carbohydrate restriction on glycemic control in adults with diabetes: A systematic review and meta-analysis.' *Diabetes Res Clin Pract.* May 2018;139:239-252.

Shai I, Schwarzfuchs D, Henkin Y, Shahar DR, Witkow S, Greenberg I, Golan R, Fraser D, Bolotin A, Vardi H, Tangi-Rozental O, et al. 'Weight loss with a low-carbohydrate, Mediterranean, or low-fat diet.' *N Engl J Med.* 2008;359(3):229-41.

Sheard NF, Clark NG, Brand-Miller JC, Franz MJ, Pi-Sunyer FX, Mayer-Davis E, Kulkarni K, Geil P. 'Dietary carbohydrate (amount and type) in the prevention and management of diabetes: a statement by the american diabetes association.' *Diabetes Care.* 2004;27(9):2266-71.

Snorgaard O, Poulsen GM, Andersen HK, Astrup A. 'Systematic review and meta-analysis of dietary carbohydrate restriction in patients with type 2 diabetes.' *BMJ Open Diabetes Res Care.* 2017;5(1):e000354.

Stern L, Iqbal N, Seshadri P, Chicano KL, Daily DA, McGrory J, Williams M, Gracely EJ, Samaha FF. 'The effects of low-carbohydrate versus conventional weight loss diets in severely obese adults: one-year follow-up of a randomized trial.' *Ann Intern Med.* 2004;140(10):778-85.

Suyoto PST. 'Effect of low-carbohydrate diet on markers of renal function in patients with type 2 diabetes: A meta-analysis.' *Diabetes Metab Res Rev.* Oct 2018;34(7):e3032.

Tay J, Luscombe-Marsh ND, Thompson CH, Noakes M, Buckley JD, Wittert GA, Yancy WS, Jr., Brinkworth GD. 'A very low-carbohydrate, low-saturated fat diet for type 2 diabetes management: a randomized trial.' *Diabetes Care.* 2014;37(11):2909-18.

Tay J, Luscombe-Marsh ND, Thompson CH, Noakes M, Buckley JD, Wittert GA, Yancy WS, Jr., Brinkworth GD. 'Comparison of low- and high-carbohydrate diets for type 2 diabetes management: a randomized trial.' *Am J Clin Nutr.* 2015;102(4):780-90.

Tay J, Thompson CH, Brinkworth GD. 'Glycemic variability: assessing glycemia differently and the implications for dietary management of diabetes.' *Annu Rev Nutr.* 2015;35:389-424.

Tay J, Thompson CH, Luscombe-Marsh ND, Noakes M, Buckley JD, Wittert GA, Brinkworth GD. 'Long-term effects of a very low carbohydrate compared with a high carbohydrate diet on renal function in individuals with type 2 diabetes: a randomized trial.' *Medicine (Baltimore).* 2015;94(47):e2181.

Tay J, Thompson CH, Luscombe-Marsh ND, Wycherley TP, Noakes M, Buckley JD, Wittert GA, Yancy WS, Jr., Brinkworth GD. 'Effects of an energy-restricted low-carbohydrate, high unsaturated fat/low saturated fat diet versus a high-carbohydrate, low-fat diet in type 2 diabetes: A 2-year randomized clinical trial.' *Diabetes Obes Metab.* Apr 2018;20(4):858-871.

Tay J, Zajac IT, Thompson CH, Luscombe-Marsh ND, Danthiir V, Noakes M, Buckley JD, Wittert GA, Brinkworth GD. 'A randomised-controlled trial of the effects of very low-carbohydrate and high-carbohydrate diets on cognitive performance in patients with type 2 diabetes.' *Br J Nutr.* 2016:1-9.

Taylor PJ, Thompson CH, Brinkworth GD. 'Effectiveness and acceptability of continuous glucose monitoring for type 2 diabetes management: A narrative review.' *J Diabetes Investig.* Jul 2018;9(4):713-725.

Taylor PJ, Thompson CH, Luscombe-Marsh ND, Wycherley TP, Wittert G, Brinkworth GD. "Efficacy of real-time continuous glucose monitoring to improve effects of a prescriptive lifestyle intervention in type 2 diabetes: a pilot study.' *Diabetes Ther.* Apr 2019;10(2):509-522.

Taylor PJ, Thompson CH, Luscombe-Marsh ND, Wycherley TP, Wittert G, Brinkworth GD, Zajac I. 'Tolerability and acceptability of real-time continuous glucose monitoring and its impact on diabetes management behaviours in individuals with type 2 diabetes – a pilot study.' *Diabetes Res Clin Pract.* Sep 2019;155:107814.

van Zuuren EJ, Fedorowicz Z, Kuijpers T, Pijl H. 'Effects of low-carbohydrate - compared with low-fat-diet interventions on metabolic control in people with type 2 diabetes: a systematic review including GRADE assessments.' *Am J Clin Nutr.* Aug 1 2018;108(2):300-331.

Westman EC, Yancy WS, Jr., Mavropoulos JC, Marquart M, McDuffie JR. 'The effect of a low-carbohydrate, ketogenic diet versus a low-glycemic index diet on glycemic control in type 2 diabetes mellitus.' *Nutr Metab (Lond).* 2008;5:36.

Witte AV, Fobker M, Gellner R, Knecht S, Floel A. 'Caloric restriction improves memory in elderly humans.' *Proc Natl Acad Sci USA.* 2009;106(4):1255-60.

Wolfe BM, Piche LA. 'Replacement of carbohydrate by protein in a conventional-fat diet reduces cholesterol and triglyceride concentrations in healthy normolipidemic subjects.' *Clin Invest Med.* 1999;22(4):140-8.

Wycherley TP, Moran LJ, Clifton PM, Noakes M, Brinkworth GD. 'Effects of energy-restricted high-protein, low-fat compared with standard-protein, low-fat diets: a meta-analysis of randomized controlled trials.' *Am J Clin Nutr.* 2012;96(6):1281-98.

Wycherley TP, Thompson CH, Buckley JD, Luscombe-Marsh ND, Noakes M, Wittert GA, Brinkworth GD. 'Long-term effects of weight loss with a very-low carbohydrate, low saturated fat diet on flow mediated dilatation in patients with type 2 diabetes: A randomised controlled trial.' *Atherosclerosis.* 2016;252:28-31.

Recipe conversion chart

Measuring cups and spoons may vary slightly from one country to another, but the difference is generally not enough to affect a recipe. All cup and spoon measures are level.

One Australian metric measuring cup holds 250 ml (8 fl oz), one Australian tablespoon holds 20 ml (4 teaspoons) and one Australian metric teaspoon holds 5 ml. North America, New Zealand and the UK use a 15 ml (3-teaspoon) tablespoon.

LENGTH

METRIC	IMPERIAL
3 mm	⅛ inch
6 mm	¼ inch
1 cm	½ inch
2.5 cm	1 inch
5 cm	2 inches
18 cm	7 inches
20 cm	8 inches
23 cm	9 inches
25 cm	10 inches
30 cm	12 inches

LIQUID MEASURES

ONE AMERICAN PINT	ONE IMPERIAL PINT
500 ml (16 fl oz)	600 ml (20 fl oz)

CUP	METRIC	IMPERIAL
⅛ cup	30 ml	1 fl oz
¼ cup	60 ml	2 fl oz
⅓ cup	80 ml	2½ fl oz
½ cup	125 ml	4 fl oz
⅔ cup	160 ml	5 fl oz
¾ cup	180 ml	6 fl oz
1 cup	250 ml	8 fl oz
2 cups	500 ml	16 fl oz
2¼ cups	560 ml	20 fl oz
4 cups	1 litre	32 fl oz

DRY MEASURES

The most accurate way to measure dry ingredients is to weigh them. However, if using a cup, add the ingredient loosely to the cup and level with a knife; don't compact the ingredient unless the recipe requests 'firmly packed'.

METRIC	IMPERIAL
15 g	½ oz
30 g	1 oz
60 g	2 oz
125 g	4 oz (¼ lb)
185 g	6 oz
250 g	8 oz (½ lb)
375 g	12 oz (¾ lb)
500 g	16 oz (1 lb)
1 kg	32 oz (2 lb)

OVEN TEMPERATURES

CELSIUS	FAHRENHEIT	CELSIUS	GAS MARK
100°C	200°F	110°C	¼
120°C	250°F	130°C	½
150°C	300°F	140°C	1
160°C	325°F	150°C	2
180°C	350°F	170°C	3
200°C	400°F	180°C	4
220°C	425°F	190°C	5
		200°C	6
		220°C	7
		230°C	8
		240°C	9
		250°C	10

Acknowledgements

First we would like to express our deep thanks to our scientific co-investigators and collaborators for their contributions to our scientific ideas and their guidance and commitment to this important research topic: Professor Manny Noakes (formerly CSIRO); Dr Jeannie Tay (formerly CSIRO and now a research scientist at the Agency for Science Technology and Research, Singapore (A-STAR)); Professor Jon Buckley (University of South Australia); Professor Gary Wittert (University of Adelaide); Professor William Yancy Jr (Duke University, USA); Professor Carlene Wilson (Flinders University); Dr Vanessa Danthiir (formerly CSIRO); Dr Ian Zajac (CSIRO) and Professor Peter Clifton (University of South Australia).

Thanks to Dr David Unwin (RCGP National Champion for Collaborative Care and Support Planning in Obesity & Diabetes – Southport, United Kingdom); Professor Katherine Samaras (Garvan Institute of Medical Research, Sydney, Australia); Dr Malcolm Riley (CSIRO); A/Prof. Beverley Mühlhäusler (CSIRO); and Dr Rob Grenfell (CSIRO), who provided their professional expertise in reviewing and advising on the book content.

A special thanks to the following individuals at the Clinical Research Team at CSIRO Health and Biosecurity for their tireless work in conducting the clinical research activities that underpin the contents of this book: Anne McGuffin, Julia Weaver and Vanessa Courage for coordinating the research trials; Janna Lutze, Dr Paul Foster, Xenia Cleanthous, Gemma Williams, Hannah Gilbert and Fiona Barr for assisting in designing and implementing the dietary interventions; Lindy Lawson, Theresa McKinnon, Rosemary McArthur and Heather Webb for their nursing expertise and clinical patient management; Vanessa Russell, Cathryn Pape, Candita Dang, Andre Nikolic and Sylvia Usher for performing biochemical assays and for other laboratory expertise; Julie Syrette and Kathryn Bastiaans for data management; Kylie Lange and Mary Barnes for assisting with statistical analyses; Bianca Frew and Asaesja Young for communications; our external fitness partners and health coaches for implementing the exercise interventions, including Luke Johnston and Annie Hastwell of Fit for Success; Kelly French, Jason Delfos, Kristi Lacey-Powell, Marilyn Woods, John Perrin, Simon Pane and Annette Beckette of South Australian Aquatic and Leisure Centre; and Angie Mondello and Josh Gniadek of Boot Camp Plus.

Thanks to the editorial and publishing team at Pan Macmillan Australia: Ingrid Ohlsson, who supported the writing of this book with great enthusiasm and encouragement; and to Ariane Durkin, Naomi van Groll and Madeleine Kane for their tireless work and support through the editorial and design process. Thanks also to editor Katri Hilden, recipe developer Tracey Pattison, recipe editor Rachel Carter, photographer Rob Palmer, stylist Emma Knowles and home economist Kerrie Ray. Lastly, thanks to the wonderful Clare Keighery for her stellar work on publicity.

Finally, and most importantly, we'd like to thank the research volunteers for their participation in our research trials. It's only through their contributions that our research and these significant advancements in clinical practices have been made possible.

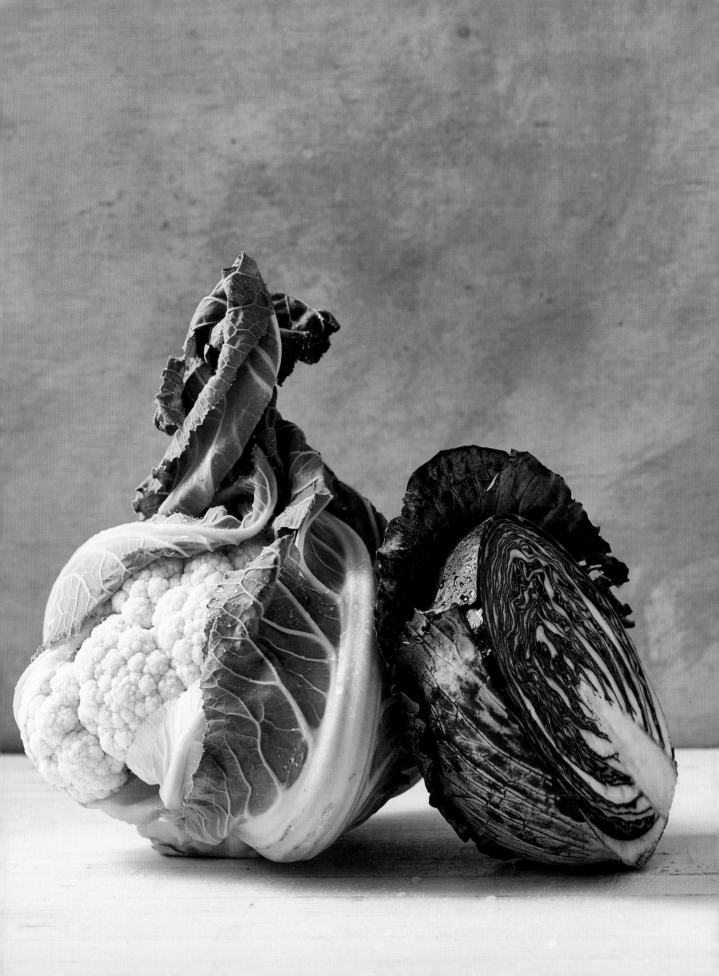

Index

First published 2020 in Macmillan
by Pan Macmillan Australia Pty Limited
Level 25, 1 Market Street, Sydney, New South Wales
Australia 2000

A CIP catalogue record for this book is available from the National Library of Australia:
http://catalogue.nla.gov.au

Design by Madeleine Kane
Recipe development by Tracey Pattison
Exercise plan by Tom Wycherley
Edited by Katri Hilden and Rachel Carter
Index by Helena Holmgren
Prop and food styling by Emma Knowles
Food preparation by Kerrie Ray
Colour + reproduction by Splitting Image Colour Studio
Printed in China by 1010 Printing International Limited

Extra photography: On page 2 (clockwise from top left) © Trinette Reed, Stocksy; Rawpixel, iStock; Nicky Lloyd, iStock; Lydia Cazorla, Stocksy; Yakobchuk Olena, iStock; Duet Postscriptum, Stocksy; Rob and Julia Campbell, Stocksy; Trent Lanz, Stocksy; Bonnin Studio, Stocksy. On page 10 (clockwise from top left) © Lordn, Shutterstock; Cameron Whitman, Stocksy; Sofie Delauw, Stocksy; Anchiy, iStock; sturti, iStock; Nadine Greeff, Stocksy; amenic181, Shutterstock; Ivan Gener, Stocksy. On page 21 © Neirfy, Creative Market. On page 24 © VikiVector, iStock; kowalska-art, iStock; A-Digit, iStock. On page 36 (clockwise from top left) © Jill Chen, Stocksy; Rob and Julia Campbell, Stocksy; Obradovic, iStock; Alto Images, Stocksy; Martí Sans, Stocksy; Rob and Julia Campbell, Stocksy; yulkapopkova, iStock; Cecilie_Arcurs, iStock. On page 42 © bsd555, iStock; Pikovit44, iStock; hakule, iStock. On page 47 © v777999, iStock; mludzen, iStock; Vikif, iStock; Serezniyf, iStock. On page 63 © Cookie Studio, Shutterstock. On page 66 (clockwise from top left) © Trinette Reed, Stocksy; olgakr, iStock; JohnnyGreig, iStock; Jill Chen, Stocksy; Trinette Reed, Stocksy; Nadine Greeff, Stocksy; Andrey Pavlov, Stocksy; Nadine Greeff, Stocksy. On page 264 (clockwise from top left) © Javier Pardina, Stocksy; Studio Firma, Stocksy; Lisovskaya, iStock; Rob and Julia Campbell, Stocksy; Mladen Zivkovic, iStock; Xsandra, iStock; PeopleImages, iStock; Lumina, Stocksy. On page 280 © Nadine Greef, Stocksy.

10 9 8 7 6 5 4 3 2 1